Autism, Spirituality, & Medical Mayhem

Dr. Patrick V. Suglia

Blue Pearl Publishing

First printing: 2017

ISBN-10: 0-692-91208-8
ISBN-13: 978-0-692-91208-9
LCCN 2017910423

Blue Pearl Publishing
1383 Pottsville Pike
Shoemakersville. PA 19555
(484) 665-2303
DrPVSuglia@Gmail.com

Edited by Rebecca M. Suglia, LCSW
Cover art designed by Shelli McVaugh

All of my thanks go to Shiva and to Muktananda who introduced me to him.

Contents

Introduction

There are four components to this book, all interwoven throughout the book. The biographical part basically picks up from where my first book, "The Doctor Is In", left off. Returning to my home town did not happen entirely by choice, and the road along the way to furthering my own cause was met with many growing pains, gains, and losses. I talk about autism not merely from a personal perspective but also from the point of view of the optimist who sees it as a serendipitous challenge. Such a point of view is not so easy unless the spirituality component is introduced. Yet, the topic of spirituality is discussed from both an evolutionary and a contemplative viewpoint. Incorporated into the picture is the largely divisive topic of specific medical practices which some people herald while others condemn.

None of the above topics are discussed lightly. Much research has been done, and references have been provided to show where the evidence came from. No matter what the subject or the debate is, the information shared in this book was meant to be timely to this day and age. Autism is no longer seen as a curse, more people are becoming interested in their own spiritual development, and, certainly, people, especially parents, are no longer taking their doctor's advice as the absolute truth when so much evidence of what is contrary is being made known. A paradigm shift has occurred, and the power is returning to the people who want the change. Although what is presented is not all-encompassing and there are many other views and subjects to be discussed, I am hoping this book becomes a tool for empowerment and encouragement and a knowledge base from which people who are awake and aware can gain strength.

1

The Unfortunate Return

April 24, 2013. My seemingly enjoyable days of being a Madman in the Desert came to a sudden and unexpected end. I left Yuma, Arizona to return to my home town of Reading, Pennsylvania to be with family. I had no choice. My hopes of becoming highly successful in my profession and to be well-off all perished in the blowing sands of the Sonoran Desert. In my first book, I tell the story of a long and winding journey of one awkward and naïve autie (person with autism) trying to make something of himself while enduring numerous health challenges, lots of bullying, and many unfair situations. When I left Reading in 1992 to find my place in this world, I embarked on a twenty-year journey that took me all across the United States. Then, after all those years, I ended up right back where I started. This time, I sported an inner strength and stamina that I otherwise never would have known had I never embarked on such a journey. And so, the story continues.

When I arrived at my mom's house four days later, there was no big welcome home celebration. There wasn't any cheering. I was "home" because I was homeless and penniless. I could have chosen to stay in a shelter in Yuma. I just might have done that if not for two things: you could only stay there ten days during any month, and you can't take a shower before 2:00 PM. Neither situation suited me because of my autistic traits and routines. Up until the day I left Yuma, I had spent most of my days staying with various friends who allowed me to live at their places temporarily. Now I had to start all over again, living with my elderly mom at the age of 51. But this was no time for shedding tears. It was a good opportunity for me to think about what I really wanted to do in life and, more importantly, how. Becoming a "doctor" just because I could and being autistic seemed to go hand in hand in setting up my eventual demise, professionally speaking. It was time to figure out what I *could* do *and* be financially successful at it. I had always been told that I was good at what I do as a chiropractor, but compliments don't pay the bills nor put food on the table. Besides, having autism meant that I was already challenged no matter what I decided on. My greatest dysfunction for all the time I had been in practice was with getting people through the door. I needed to come up with a different plan.

The small town of Bowmansville, located twelve miles south of my home town of Reading, was just what I needed for my peace of mind. My parents had bought a home there in 2003 because they wanted to get away from the city after their retirement. The relaxing farmland of the Pennsylvania Dutch countryside was ideal. But first, they took a detour to the Florida Keys. The six months I spent in Florida living with them between 2000 and 2002 was beneficial to me when I was between failed business ventures. Once they moved to Bowmansville, I felt at ease whenever I came back to PA to visit. I certainly preferred the sound of a passing horse and buggy to the bustling of heavy traffic. The quietude of the country contributed to the restful state I felt overall even though I regretted having to live there at that point of my life. Bowmansville was just a place where I could pull myself together before moving on to my next venture. Despite all

I'd been through, I still had no intention of staying in the area, let alone in Pennsylvania.

Part of my re-collecting I had to do entailed flashing back to a lot of old "stuff" that was still in my brain, mostly memories of events that made me eager for something better. One day when I was in my mid-20s, my dad said to me, "I don't know what it is with you. Everywhere you go you seem to end up having problems!" Surely, I was very aware of this. But I was a good person, so it couldn't have been my fault. I figured the world is just full of nitwits, and my slowness just meant that anything that had to be accomplished would take a lot of effort. Knowing that this was just the way life was for me is what kept me going, often accompanied by much frustration and deep despair. I kept telling myself it would all turn around eventually.

Although no turnaround ever presented itself, the road certainly became much more bearable after I was diagnosed with PDD-NOS, a component of the autism spectrum, at the age of 45. Not only did I now have an explanation for all my difficulties but I suddenly became friends with many other adults at various autism support groups whom all shared similar stories of rejection and hardship. The diagnosis also took the edge off an already-frayed marriage, which I eventually brought to an end anyway. I finally realized that I would never be able to satisfy a person who could never identify exactly how it was that I was causing her dissatisfaction even after almost ten years of marriage.

At the time of my diagnosis, I was living in Minnesota. There, I had plenty of opportunities to connect and to share my story. The adult support group at the Autism Society of Minnesota was quite large, and I connected well with most of the people there. Simply being around them automatically gave me a sense of camaraderie. Words did not have to be shared, and they often weren't. On occasion, I would receive an invite to be part of a panel or discussion group where professionals and caregivers could ask questions about what life is like on the autism spectrum. Since I already enjoyed getting up in front of audiences to teach in various community education programs, I put together a three-hour presentation (which I turned into a four-hour presentation after returning to Pennsylvania) about what it's like to live with autism. It felt rewarding to finally meet people who actually listened to what I have to say and who finally gave me the credibility I felt I deserved.

Although things seemed to have swung in a positive direction at the time, both lack of professional success and the need to get out of a dead-end marriage led me to eventually leave Minnesota. That's how I ended up in Arizona in the first place. I figured the beauty and the heat of southwestern Arizona would benefit me. But it wasn't just a whim that took me there. It was an astrocartograph, an astrologically-based map of planetary influences. The astrocartograph hinted that anywhere along my Jupiter line was where I would be sure to enjoy my greatest professional successes. It just so happened that Yuma was the furthest south I could go within the United States along that line. The plan might have actually worked the way I anticipated had everything panned out the way I thought it would. All I needed was a little more time and a lot more money. After spending only ten months in Yuma, I had to go home, even though home never really *felt* like "home."

So, here I was right back where I started. Two decades had passed, and it all seemed just as indifferent as it was before. Sure, the countryside and the scenery of Pennsylvania are beautiful. But I never felt as though there was an opportunity for me to evolve here. People treated me as though I was either insignificant or a bother. Even all the years I spent offering my time to the volunteer ambulance and fire companies seemed to have gone unnoticed. During that point in my life, though, my involvement with the ambulance and fire companies was my *entire* life. There was nothing else, even though I knew deep down inside that I was capable of so much more. Fast forward twenty-and-a-half years, and here I was again. This time, I had so much more life experience including having been married, achieving a doctorate degree from the largest and best chiropractic college in the world, and having been given the great gift of spiritual awakening from an authentic Indian guru. I was different now, no longer a less-than-average joe. Since it seemed that I was in for a long stay, it was time to find out if my home town was any different.

Despite the successes I did experience during the twenty-plus years I was away, I didn't have much to show for it. Just because one is educated and has a lot of experience in various areas doesn't mean he's going to be financially well-off or even stable. I was far from stable. Throughout my entire adult life, I never really was financially stable except for during the thirteen months, from November 1992 until December 1993, that I worked as a Respiratory Therapist in Valparaiso, Indiana. In September 2001, when I left my job as an associate chiropractor to open my own practice at a truck stop in the Pocono Mountains, I brought to an end a brief period of stability that lasted only four months. Because I was back in a state of lack, I lived in my office. I slept on an air mattress that I inflated each night and then tucked away under my desk during the day. I had my own private shower, something I never could have done without. Nine months afterward, I got married. During my entire marriage, I never made more than a four-figure income. When I first moved to Arizona, I survived for the first three months on the little bit of money my dad gave me before I left. The rest of the time I lived on the pocket change I made from seeing the few patients I had and on the goodness of other people. Then the ride was over.

Roughly 6% of all homeless people in America have a college degree[1], and only about 24% of all people with autism have any kind of employment whatsoever[2]. Keeping right in line with these figures, it was always a major challenge for me to find and keep employment for any significant amount of time. It was nearly impossible for me to build a clientele as a chiropractor or as a holistic healer. Being back in Pennsylvania was certainly not going to make any difference, I felt. After all, professional woes are why I left in the first place. But once again, I had my work cut out for me. I not only needed to get myself back on my feet again but I also had the challenge of getting my unforgiving family off my back.

During the first two months of being home, my priority was to finish writing my first book, a project I had worked diligently on half the time I lived in Arizona. After receiving more than sixty rejection letters from traditional publishers, I went ahead and published it myself as a print-on-demand project. I then spent the rest of the summer sending out resume upon resume and application after application. I applied for every kind of job I could stand to do, such as office work or being a security guard. I even went out of my comfort zone and applied for dishwashing and janitorial jobs. Most of my resumes and inquiries went unanswered. For the rare interview I did manage to land, usually for some menial work, I endured the usual stress that a person with autism faces. Many adults with autism never get the chance to prove themselves in the work setting because of poor interviewing skills which cause them to strike out before they ever get a chance[3]. I was very well aware of this from much personal experience. But I had to do *something* to appease the naysayers and those who thought I was lazy and uncaring. I also figured I might just get lucky somewhere, somehow.

Most of my summer was uneventful. If I wasn't at home filling out job applications, I was taking walks around the development where my mom and I lived. I stayed at home to keep my mom company most of the time. After the initial disappointment over having to return home, I felt happy to be there for my mom, to be of help to her and to do errands for her. Ever since my dad passed away from a chronic condition in June of 2012, life just wasn't the same for her. My parents had been married for fifty-six years, and they were both in their late 70s. With my older brother, Damon, living almost fifty miles away and my younger brother, Peter, a hundred miles away, I felt obliged, willingly, to stick around and be close to home just in case anything would happen to my mom. It was a win-win situation despite the obvious tension caused by my lack of an income.

As the end of summer approached, I started getting the bug to leave again. I figured if I'm going to struggle, I may as well do it someplace I might have a chance to succeed. My home town wasn't it. Turning once again to the astrocartograph, I figured I'd look for opportunities along my Venus line, as suggested by my Reiki Master, Betty McKeon. Venus represents life successes, including money, springing forth out of romantic interests. Although romance was never a primary motivator for me, I thought living along the Venus line just might prove to be where I finally enjoy success *and* feel at home. It made things quite interesting when I discovered there is only one part of one U.S. state my Venus line passes through, and that is the far eastern tip of Maine. I then started looking for work in Maine as well as locally. My new intention was to save up enough money to make the trip up to and to become licensed to practice in Maine. Maine was no stranger to me. I was there more than once during the summers between 1977 and 1981 while visiting my Uncle Valent who lived in the Ossipee Mountains of New Hampshire.

For the two-and-a-half-month period between leaving Minnesota in April 2012 and moving to Arizona, I had returned to Pennsylvania to help take care of my ailing dad. Just a few days before he passed away, he said something that made a world of difference in our relationship. As I was growing up, he couldn't stand the fact that I was a sensitive and laid back introvert and philosopher. I was much too nice. His goal was to turn me into a "man" by getting tough on me psychologically and sometimes physically. He referred to it as his way of using "reverse psychology" to motivate me. I always saw it as his affirmation of disapproval, and perhaps disgust, that I wasn't living up to his standards. Now, in his weakened state, he said to me, "If we had known back then that you had autism, I would have done things differently." It seemed that my dad finally understood that I had challenges and difficulties. I figured it finally dawned on him why I always ended up having problems wherever I went. He then apologized for all the meanness and condescending talk. I told him that I understood where he was coming from. At this point, I figured that if he had been any softer on me, I would not have developed the strengths that I *did* have. In that moment, he became the only member of my family to truly understand what it's like to have autism.

2

A Turning Point

Spring turned into summer, and summer turned into fall. Nothing ever changed. One day was just like the previous day. That's the way it stayed for 156 days. Then, during the evening of October 1, everything changed. Thanks to my Aunt Rosemarie (my dad's sister) doing a little promoting of my first book to her husband Eugene's second cousin Donna, Donna ended up recommending it to her niece Becky. Becky was the owner of a multi-practitioner wellness center in Kutztown called U3 (pronounced "You Cubed"): Body, Mind, & Spirit. Donna figured I might make a good fit for Becky's business. At 8:12 PM, I received an email from Becky. She inquired as to whether or not I'd be interested in working at her wellness center. I called her right away, and we set up an interview for the next afternoon. What resulted was something far greater than what I, Becky, or her two business partners ever anticipated.

I learned that I was not interviewing for a paid position. Instead, this was a way for me to become associated with like-minded people whereby we could market ourselves together as a team. I was happy with that since I didn't know of any fellow natural healers in the area. Any way I could get myself out there was fine with me. Fears of being interviewed in the traditional sense quickly vanished when I realized this was anything but a typical interview. Everyone was so relaxed and informal, and they did all the listening.

Even though I had neither intention nor enough money to renew my license to practice chiropractic in Pennsylvania, advertising "structural alignment" as a softer alternative to chiropractic and Reiki healing seemed enough to classify myself as a Holistic Healer. All I had to do was demonstrate what I do and to explain my philosophy on healing. Becky and her partners were all very impressed not just with my views but with the gentleness and effectiveness of the Reiki and structural alignment care I demonstrated. They were all quite thrilled and excited to add me to their team.

I was having quite an amazing day, and the best was yet to come. My time at the wellness center eventually led to something quite unexpected and serendipitous. At one point, we were all sitting on the sofa in the reception area. I was speaking intently and enthusiastically about spiritual awareness and evolution. Because of my intuitive gift of clairsentience, that is keen perceptiveness to the flow of etheric energy, I noticed something rather peculiar with Becky. The more I spoke, the more her attention changed. She was no longer looking at me as just a potential business associate. She began contemplating a romantic interest. Although I felt flattered, I felt a bit uneasy about how quickly such feelings came about. Her energy emanated like a blasting stereo. I never felt anyone's energy quite so strongly and loud. It was as if a giant wave of electricity was making its way around the room. That's about the best way I can describe what it felt like.

In reality, this is what it feels like whenever I pick up on energies. What made this encounter with Becky particularly interesting is how powerful a blast it was. Clairsentient people are keenly and consciously aware of this energy, and they know what it is saying to them. Energy waves can feel like either electrical charges, changes in temperature, or sudden feelings of urgency or calmness as the case may be. For most people, this all happens subconsciously such as when one has a "bad feeling" about a particular person or situation. For the clairsentient, it's as if the mind itself, or a spirit, is placing images in the mind when certain waves are felt. Some may say, "You are an empath." But the main difference between an empath and a clairsentient, according to Alex Myles, author of *The Empath*, is that while empaths can feel emotions and energies in their immediate surroundings, clairsentients can pick up on a person's thoughts and even sense distant energies and events. My clairsentient abilities only became stronger after I was trained in Reiki and started meditating regularly. It's been my compass when caring for patients and making life choices ever since.

During the course of the interview, the business partners lied on my table to receive a sample of my healing work. Just before it was Becky's turn, I pulled her aside and asked her to tone down her energy. She was astonished to discover that I was able to sense it. I can say, with certainty, that even though autism has hampered my ability to read body language throughout the years, this uncanny intuition has always saved the day. Becky wasn't quite able to contain her energy blasts, even though she tried. After talking to her for some time after the interview, we agreed to go out on a date after U3's upcoming open house the following Sunday. During the next four days, Becky and I chatted a tremendous amount both online and by phone. We grew more and more ecstatic about our upcoming date. We became so confident in our connection that we were certain we would make a great pair.

The following Sunday was October 6. It was a day of affirmation for two major reasons. First, after having cared for all the people at U3's open house in the ways that I did, I felt as though I was at home professionally. I was indeed doing what I was *meant* to do in life; I am a healer by calling. It felt extremely rewarding to be in that role again and to be busy doing it. I am at my best when caring for somebody, and not in an egoistic way. Pinpointing someone's needs accurately, whether through examination or intuition, proved my natural ability and proficiency in doing so. Making the necessary corrections and giving the appropriate advice seemed to happen effortlessly and without much thought. The second affirmation was that Becky and I were definitely compatible beyond expectations. We were suddenly in a relationship that needed no preambles or introductions. It just *was*. And now between my involvement with U3 and my relationship with Becky, life suddenly looked brighter and definitely more promising than it had in many years. I suddenly had a reason to stay right where I was.

Even though I still wasn't making any money, I at least had something to do. A goal and a plan were in place. I spent time in Kutztown walking around marketing myself and U3. Also, I now had a significant other to spend time with. Although my introverted nature produced the same ol' same ol' while talking to people in the town, things were more bearable having Becky with her extroverted nature by my side. Even though my job search continued, I no longer planned on moving off to Maine. A door had opened that I didn't want to close. While I continued to spend my usual weekdays with my mom, I spent my weekends with Becky at her house in Hamburg. Becky, her mom, and her eighteen-year-old daughter Brittany had signed the lease on the house they lived in just days after Becky and I met. After the passing of Becky's second husband in December 2011 and her dad just three months before the move, she and her mom could no longer afford to live in the semidetached houses where they had lived next door to each other in Tamaqua, twenty-four miles further north.

Visiting the town of Hamburg was endearing to me. I had fond memories of that place. When I was a kid, my dad would take me to work with him at the former Algonquin Chemical Company. During the late 80s and early 90s, I'd make regular visits, usually with my parents, to Jack DiMaio's restaurant, which is now located in Orwigsburg. The annual King Frost parade on the last Saturday in October was another good memory from when I was in the high school marching band and, in later years, as a Fire Police officer directing traffic. I had also worked at the former Ames Department Store setting up display fixtures before it first opened for business in late 1986. Hamburg seemed to be the last small town of Berks County, PA, where family life is important, crime is low, and people still had values.

Since things were going so well at that time, between showing signs of life professionally and having a great relationship, I figured I'd bring Becky home to meet mom. My mom seemed to like Becky from what I told her, most of all the fact that she understood my impoverished state. After all, Becky was not much better off herself, financially speaking. We made plans to go to my mom's house for dinner the last Monday in October after spending the weekend together. While at U3 that Monday afternoon, I received a phone call from our neighbor. She called to tell me that she had to take my mom to the hospital the previous day. Apparently, years of suffering from medication-induced liver failure finally caught up with her, and she suddenly could no longer function independently. Her problem had originated as an acquired blood infection. Because of her other health issues, she slowly and steadily declined. Instead of us enjoying an evening with mom at home, Becky and I visited her in the hospital. My mom spent the following whole week in the hospital. I brought Becky there once again to visit her. That's when my mom said to me, "She's a very nice girl."

Over the next few weeks, it became apparent that my mom's condition would not improve. During the same period of time, I continued to spend more time with Becky and her daughter in Hamburg and at the U3 office in Kutztown. My mom eventually decided that she just wanted to give up and leave this world. She wanted to go to the other side to be with my dad. She spent the last two weeks of her life in hospice care. The day before she passed away, she asked me how I was doing. I assured her she had nothing to worry about. I didn't say that just to put her mind at ease. I sincerely believed, for the first time since ending my marriage in April 2012, that I would fare out well despite my current hardships. I now had Becky and her family, who gave me more encouragement and credibility than I had received from anyone since my days of being a student chiropractor. Becky and I figured that if things continued to improve, and if they kept going in the direction they were, we would end up living together permanently.

During the early morning hours of December 1, my mom passed away. Several years of physical pain and suffering finally came to an end. Now my brothers and I turned our attention to cleaning out the house in Bowmansville and preparing for it to be sold. With Damon having power of attorney, he was the one calling the shots. It also became unclear as to where I would live when the time came for me to leave. Becky was living in an already-full house with her daughter and her mom. The only other option available was to live in the home of my Aunt Rosemarie downtown. Aunt Rosemarie no longer lived there, but two of her children did. Those two never talked to each other, and there was a lot of animosity between them. That was a situation better avoided, so I wasn't very fond of that option. That option would have me sleeping in a cold basement with the only working bathroom on the main floor of the house. Even though it was better than being completely homeless, I still hoped for something better.

I expected to be gone from my mom's house by the end of December. Needless to say, I was full of angst now for two reasons. Losing my mom and the roof over my head in the same month would be devastating. That didn't happen, though. I continued to stay at the house for the time being. The cleanout process and contacting a realtor were taking a very long time. During this time, I applied for public assistance since it was apparent that I wouldn't be working anywhere anytime soon. I also needed to get back to taking anticoagulant medication for my prosthetic heart valve since I had not been taking it for more than a year at that point. I was also not under the care of any cardiologist. I was living on a wing and a prayer, but that was certainly nothing new.

Damon made me aware of the arrangements that mom and dad had made in their will that directly affected me. Although my parents had divided their money into thirds between us brothers, my third was not made directly available to me. It was placed in a trust account for two reasons: so that it could not be garnished by any creditors, and because they felt I was too irresponsible to manage money. Damon was placed in charge of the trust, and the trust could only be tapped into with his permission and for emergency situations only. Looking at it from a different perspective, I apparently would still be without self-supporting funds including the money I would have needed to renew my license to practice as a chiropractor in Pennsylvania. It took more than a year before I even had the courage to ask my brother for my money for that purpose. When I finally did in January 2015, Damon said, "It may seem unfair that mom and dad didn't give you your share outright. But if it's going to go toward helping you succeed in life, I'll allow you to have money for that." I eventually learned that I would be given an annual allotment of $3,000 (before taxes), and the first would be given to me in January.

The holidays were certainly a rollercoaster time for me. Despite the downslide with the loss of my mom and the potential loss of a place to live, there was also the upswing with the strengthening of a wonderful relationship and an increase in the number of clientele I took care of, thanks to Becky and U3. There was yet another coincidentally serendipitous state of affairs brewing during this time. At the exact same time Becky and I started dating, Becky's mom Pam started dating a man named Ken. Ken was actually an old family friend, and Pam and Ken had reconnected recently after they both lost their spouses during the previous ten months. They were there for each other at the right time, and their togetherness was blossoming into something more than just a friendship. As the end of the year approached, Pam and Ken started making plans to get married the next summer. Once married, Pam would live with Ken at his place in nearby Windsor Castle. Then, starting in August, the house in Hamburg would have enough room in it for me to move into. I felt better knowing that wherever I ended up after leaving my mom's house would be only a temporary stay should Becky and I remain in the fantastic relationship we were enjoying.

Since I was all by myself while staying at my mom's house, and U3 and Becky's house were more than thirty miles away, I started spending much more time at Becky's place in Hamburg. I would return to my mom's house in Bowmansville for only one or two nights during the week. Becky's family was glad for my company, and I helped them with chores around the house. Pam and Ken eventually decided they were going to take a road trip across the United States in June, and they would get married at a chapel in Las Vegas. They also planned for Pam to start living with Ken *before* they left on their trip. This announcement came as welcome news to everyone. My planned move-in date was suddenly moved up by two months. But then there was yet another change that seemed to put a damper on things. Damon decided that mom's house should be cleaned out by the end of March, which meant that I would have to be gone then too.

One final day was planned for us brothers and our families to get together for the final move. That day was March 12. An auction house that Damon contacted came to take every last bit of furniture except for what us brothers wanted to keep for ourselves. By mid-afternoon, the place was bare, down to the walls. Becky came with a friend who had a pickup truck to take the sectional sofa that filled the TV room. That sofa was where my dad spent most his free time and where my mom took her naps every afternoon. It was the only item from the house that I kept, along with one of my dad's computer printers. Later in the day, I left the house in Bowmansville for the last time. Becky's home in Hamburg was now my home. Although Pam did not yet live with Ken, she was okay with me moving in early since it was only a short time before she would be moving out. Also, they enjoyed having me there as I was already very much a part of their family.

Cohabiting with Becky added a whole new challenge to my life. It's important to not associate the word "challenge" with "difficulty" or "adversity." I experienced many things in my life, mostly rejection, bullying, aloneness, disapproval by loved ones, disapproval by coworkers, and plenty of physical illness. But now things have changed. I was living with a person who accepted me and loved me despite all the reasons why others avoided me. That spoke volumes of the type of woman I now had in my life. After all, she had difficulties of her own over the years, and she was just as happy to finally be with somebody who understood her and who "gets" her. Acceptance was something new to both of us, and our mutual challenge was for each of us to get used to it. Our relationship deepened and solidified quickly, mostly due to similarities in our life paths and goals and in how spiritually compatible we were.

There was yet another component to the new relationship. I not only had a significant other who I clicked with extraordinarily well but I also had to adjust to being around her teenage daughter. Brittany added a whole new dimension to the challenge. When I was her age, I was in the throes of my naïveté and introversion. I had no idea how to communicate with someone her age. At first, she wasn't all that accepting because my autistic tendencies tried her patience. She couldn't stand how detail-oriented I was with many things, especially daily bathroom and kitchen routines. She found it difficult to hear me at times because of my low voice volume. What ended up happening was that I would elicit the same condescending responses I usually received from people when I was her age. After some time, and after some explaining of what autism is from both me and Becky, Brittany became more tolerant.

With Becky being a social worker by profession, she had great experience dealing with people who have all kinds of disabilities. Knowing this gave me a level of comfort I never had with my first wife. Becky's level of acceptance and understanding was also unprecedented. In due time, Brittany became quite accepting and loving as well. Because of the change in her outlook, I found it easier to communicate with her and to explain myself. Once we jumped over this rather benign bump in the road, our relationship grew to a level not commonly found in one between a daughter and her mom's boyfriend, one in which we found common grounds in science fact and fiction, and also in our uncanny geekiness. Perhaps the greatest perk to come from this new and odd relationship was my sudden fandom of the British sci-fi adventure Doctor Who.

During the early months of living with Becky, I continued to develop my business plan. My clientele grew somewhat due to placing coupons on daily deal websites. In July of 2014, my brother gave me some extra money to replace my oil-guzzling station wagon after it was damaged in an accident. With that money, I bought a minivan my brother had picked out. That minivan became my actual office which I used to make house calls. I also continued to promote my writing works at various presentations and book signings. Despite what seemed like an upturn in professional success, the monetary income was still stagnant. 2014 was a year of living on medical assistance, food stamps, and the good-heartedness of a girlfriend who was in the exact same boat. While Becky was slightly better off with regular private clients and a low-paying job, I contributed the best I could by caring for the house and by being there when Becky and Brittany needed help with something. It was good to have a "family" of my own to take care of, and it felt wonderful to be loved and appreciated in return. After all, if the positive trend were to continue, in time they really would be my family.

3

What Sets Me Apart

When I became a chiropractor in March of 2000, I hadn't a clue of the difficulty I was about to face trying to build a practice, trying to attract clientele, in the real world. Not being able to do so adequately as an intern was part of the reason why I graduated from chiropractic school eighteen months after I originally planned to. With the financial support of my dad over the years, I was able to go here and there to open this office or try that idea. Nothing ever worked out. Of course, at that time I didn't know I had autism. Nor did I have a definitive label, INFJ, on my profusely introverted nature. And, of course, neither my dad nor my wife at the time, who were both losing their patience very quickly, knew why I struggled so much. My experience with marketing, in my own view, was that a person's first impression of me as I approached them was that I am a weak or insignificant person, a nuisance who is wasting both our times trying to sell something my intended audience couldn't care less about.

Dr. Temple Grandin, a world-renowned autism advocate and fellow autie, addresses the need for people with autism to create a portfolio that displays their strengths since one of the greatest weaknesses of people with autism is verbal interaction. I didn't start using a portfolio, though, until I was living in Arizona. The portfolio contained an explanation of all my chiropractic techniques and skills. It also contained all my accomplishments and credentials dating back through all the years I've been in health care. If I did somehow end up striking someone's interest, I let my portfolio do the talking for me. In the end, though, I still ended up with nothing. It seemed I lost people mainly at the disclosure of the fact that I had autism.

Along with the portfolio, I felt the need to explain why I was so different from the rest, which I came to realize as a vital marketing strategy for *any* business. Every entrepreneur has his or her own "something different" to offer from the next person. The customer or client simply needs to find somebody that he or she clicks well with. When it comes to the world of holistic or "alternative" healers, there are many out there who all seem to be doing the same thing. I often hear the complaints of people who had to go to many different people before they found someone who could help them. In reality, this is just the way it is. Not everyone will use the same techniques, and not everyone will stand by the same philosophy behind their work.

Some people wonder what it is that sets me apart from the rest of the pack. I usually don't mention these things other than the obvious of my office being on wheels. It comes down to experiences, skills, and knowledge that others *might* not have which give me unique perspective and insight. But it is also the *gift* of being both on the autism spectrum and having an INFJ Myers-Briggs personality type that allows what appears oblivious to others to appear as clear as day to me. When you combine the rather-profound level of introspection that is inherent with autism with the introversion of the INFJ personality type, the details of the outside world tend to stand out more, and they undergo greater assimilation and scrutiny. This is a second-nature process for someone who has been doing this since the day he was born.

Probably the first and foremost feature that sets me apart is that I can identify on a personal level with my clients and patients who have deeply-rooted chronic conditions. Before ever making my debut in the world of health care in 1982, I had been through so much of my own health crises, and I continued to experience them over the years. The pain from chronic ear infections and kidney stone attacks, the fear surrounding having open heart surgery and cardiac ablation, the mystery surrounding a 14-1/2-year battle with Chronic Fatigue Syndrome, and two devastating bouts of food poisoning, just to name a few of my challenges, all provided me with great lessons in tolerance and empathy. The Chronic Fatigue Syndrome existed during most of my time as a student chiropractor and for much of my first marriage. It was certainly disheartening to live most days unable to think clearly and feeling as though I was wearing a suit of lead. That was the story of my life between April 1995 and October 2009. It is mind-boggling the things that go through your head during the hours upon hours you spend lying in bed when you're unable to move any further than the edge of the bed. It's also interesting to hear the words of family, the ones you'd think should care the most, when they tell you you're just making it all up. I know what all this is like. Because of it, I can relate better with those who seek my help.

Another thing that sets me apart from most of the crowd is that I am, after all, a chiropractor. Much of the general population has no idea what a chiropractor does nor what it takes to become one. There is a reason why chiropractors are called "doctor." Becoming one requires eight years (minimum) of education, just like any other type of doctor.

We learn the same basic sciences as a medical or osteopathic physician but with much more emphasis or neuroanatomy and physiology rather than pharmaceutical and surgical treatments. After all, chiropractic has much more to do with keeping the entire body working at its optimum potential than merely "popping bones." We go through a rigorous internship where we take care of actual patients under supervision in a clinic or preceptorship program for at least two years. We have regulating boards, both national and state level, whose exams we need to pass in order to become licensed to practice after we graduate.

I've heard more than one M.D. who attended chiropractic school say, "This is a whole lot tougher than I thought!", and they struggled the whole way through the program. It really isn't easy. Thus, I frown a whole lot upon those fellow chiropractors who make us into either clowns with their unprofessional behavior or gimmicks and also those who make us look like glorified physical therapists with their roller tables, zapping machines, and waterbeds. To me, both groups miss the whole point of becoming a chiropractor in the first place. Neither selling vitamins, oils, putting people on machines, massage, nor physical therapy have anything to do with what chiropractic *really* is.

There are so many named adjusting techniques used by chiropractors to help realign the bones of the body, some which are forceful in nature and others which hardly use any motion at all. As for my preference, I feel I am being most effective, and my patients agree, when I focus on studying the biomechanics of the body as a whole before proceeding to use the bones as fulcrums and levers to make corrections where and when needed. Much of what I do is based on a technique known as the Thompson Drop Table

Technique. However I never follow a recipe approach to deciding on how I'm going to correct a structural misalignment or subluxation (bone misalignment that is impinging upon a nerve's normal function).

There are other techniques I use. But, first and foremost, I always follow my instincts through observation of each individual's patterns of movement as I examine one's entire skeletal framework. Most people are on my table, being cared for by hand alone, for about twenty minutes. In contrast, many chiropractors may keep a patient on the table for roughly three minutes as they go through a cookbook analysis or may even use machinery in lieu of actually placing their hands on a person to make an adjustment. Chiropractic involves the moving of bones *only*, either by hand or with a hand-operated adjusting instrument. All else is fluff.

In August of 2012, I reached my thirtieth year of involvement in the health care field. It all began when I became an ambulance attendant, volunteering for the Governor Mifflin Area Ambulance Association in Shillington, PA. The lifesaving heart surgery I had at the age of nineteen left me unable to be a firefighter any longer, yet I was still allowed to be active with Emergency Medical Services squads. That switch set the course for the rest of my life. During those fantastic years working with the ambulance and paramedic crews, I witnessed many gut-wrenching situations which only strengthened me after I learned how to deal with such events. One thing that made me especially sought-after was the fact that my short stature automatically made me the go-to person when someone was needed to crawl into tight spots to rescue someone. As I started contemplating a career in health care in the beginning, I first worked as a nurse aid while spending a year in nursing school. Ultimately, I became a Respiratory Therapist. That was my profession until I left the world of mainstream medicine behind in December of 1993. That's when I moved to Atlanta, Georgia to attend chiropractic school.

My medical training surely came in handy as it became the foundation upon which I built my knowledge and abilities in other fields of healing. This is certainly a plus, to have such a core experience which many fellow chiropractors and natural healers never had exposure to. Knowing exactly what medicine has to offer and what the alternatives can do gives me an edge that most others do not have. I feel dismayed when my counterparts attempt to pooh-pooh medicine. I am equally as frustrated when those in medicine think that all Complementary and Alternative Medicine (CAM) therapies are baseless and quackery. Because I've been trained in healing arts on both sides of the fence, I know exactly where to draw the line. I know what I can take care of with chiropractic and with Reiki. I also know very well when it's time to refer someone to a medical practitioner.

My training in Reiki healing is yet another thing that sets me apart. I'm not just talking about *any* Reiki. I'm talking specifically about traditional Usui Reiki as Taught by Takata. This is *not* the New-Age stuff that most people in the United States are doing these days. It is *not* holding my hands above a person or waving them around, calling upon spirit guides and angels. Just about *every* person I ever did Reiki on, since I was trained in the 2nd degree of it in November 1998, told me that what they experienced from me was far more beneficial to them than any type of energy healing they had received before. Reiki works on all three levels of existence, that is physical, psychological, and spiritual. My Reiki training from Betty helped me to cognize what the word "healing" means in a multidimensional way.

This type of Reiki is like a focused laser that really can be felt through the hands of one who has been trained in the "as Taught by Takata" method. What I find interesting, however, is that there are Reiki practitioners out there who staunchly believe they are practicing this method yet they do quite the opposite from the methods and against the principles Takata taught. I've even been approached by these practitioners over the years with questions after they realized that what I do is very different. This doesn't make other forms of Reiki bogus or ineffective. Every type helps in some way. But just as in chiropractic, one should really know what technique or method they are using and not confuse it with something else.

Also, thanks to Betty, I received the greatest gift anyone on a spiritual quest could possibly receive, and that is Shaktipat, or the awakening of the inner Kundalini energy. To the lay person, this may mean nothing. But to someone who considers him or herself a spiritual seeker, this means *everything*. When you have received Shaktipat from a true guru, and you keep the fire alive through spiritual practice, you *automatically* see past the mere physical façade of a person or an event, and you are connected with the comprising essence, the consciousness, behind it all. It is important to keep in mind that the Shaktipat experience is not to be confused with a religious belief or practice. Nor is it to be passed off as an imaginary occurrence or a strange dream. It is a spiritual experience that a person from any religious tradition can have. I will talk more about the significance of Shaktipat and about the spiritual journey later in this book.

During the years that both autism and my severely-introverted personality type kept me quiet and naïve, I was unknowingly building an inner strength, an uncanny ability to see elephants in the room and to see through the fog. When I spoke, I had something profound to say. However, when I tried to speak merely to be sociable, I proved myself to be a bumbling idiot. While I can still be a bumbling idiot on any given day, one thing is for certain — I was made to be a healer. Although I've come a long way, I still have a lot to learn. No one ever really stops learning. You can get good at what you do by developing a system that works for you, as I have. But you continuously get better when you always keep your mind open for the next learning opportunity. The "healer" who tells me that he has *the* answer is the buffoon I pay no attention to. Every person is here to be of service to someone else or to something greater than his or her own self. The day you stop learning is the day God calls you from this life. Until then, education is a continuum, as are change and spiritual evolution. Conscious awareness of these truths at all times sets me apart.

4

The Eight Spiritual Laws of Success

Those who have known me from about the age of thirty onward know very well about my struggles and about my travels here and there, trying to be professionally successful. When redefining success to account for what one accomplishes in life as opposed to how much money one earns, it becomes apparent that I have always been quite successful at just about everything I set out to do. The journey had indeed been marred by my social ineptitude and the necessity of much repetition in learning new tasks. These are the most obvious outward observations one can make to be assured that I am challenged. Although being able to afford one's own roof over his head and food on his table as a result of his own efforts is ideal, this should never be part of one's measure of success.

During the last week of September 2014, I was gifted with eight intuitively-inspired rules for professional success. I think they were meant to be words of wisdom directed at me, given my ongoing and obvious struggles. Both building a clientele and attracting the wrong type of people were unending woes. These rules suddenly started popping into my head after I paid a visit to my parents' grave. I do believe that we receive inspiration from those who have passed on, yet I found the timing to be quite coincidental since my parents were never very "spiritual" per se, albeit somewhat open-minded. I found these rules to dig quite deep, hitting on inner beliefs rather than on outer-world circumstances. Some of them were merely hard lessons learned over time that needed to be made part of my conscience. I am sharing them here along with my commentaries because I know they can be of benefit to anyone.

1. Never overinflate your own importance, especially if this leads you to trying to impress others.

I find it unfortunate that many people do what they do, especially in the holistic healing field, simply because it's a good way for them to put themselves on a pedestal. People like this may build a huge clientele because they possess good marketing skills. But the ones who can see right through them will avoid them like the plague. In his audio CD "The Power of Intention," the late Dr. Wayne Dyer states, "Let go of self-importance. It's your ego at work." When you think that what you do is about proving yourself somehow or about making yourself look superior in some way, you will eventually fall hard and suffer greatly. Karma doesn't allow masks to be worn for very long. Playing the role of the expert or the healer in a loud and perhaps obnoxious way is how many people actually try to cover up a deeply-rooted lack — lack of esteem, confidence, and sense of purpose.

Throughout my travels, I often found that people who proclaim they are the "best" at something are really the ones who do the most harm. They find it easy to compensate, though, because of the volume of their own horn. In contrast, I often found the authentic healer to be the one you find when your quest is true. That healer probably won't be doing much advertising, and he might even have a small, quaint practice. Such healers are not focused primarily on bringing droves of people through their door. They know they have nothing to prove. They value the time they spend with their patients and clients. They measure their success in quality, not quantity. Their aim is truly to help a person heal, not to impress or to make a name for themselves. This same principle applies to people of any profession, not just healers. The most honest deeds come from the person whose main intent is to be of service, not from the one who is self-serving.

2. The moment you hold hands with your own ego is the moment you stop experiencing the greatness of God's love working through you. Get yourself out of the way!

Have you ever heard someone say, with true sincerity, that they are a natural at something or that they were inspired to create or do something fantastic? Such instinctive works are the result of the Divine's presence within us. In the words of St. Francis of Assisi, "Lord, make me a channel of your peace," it is important to keep in mind the key word "*channel*." A channel is a conduit through which something passes. Not unlike any one of us, St. Francis was that. The Divine does its great works *through* us. For that to happen, though, we have to open the channel. We do this simply by bowing to the greatness and the will of the Divine. We humble ourselves, thereby turning any credit due and any opinion of the mind that may get in the way over to the Source, which we are connected to. Thoughts, adversities, and the need to take the credit are all products of the ego, that is, the sense that you are the doer. In reality, you are not the doer.

Being given honors, promotions, and rewards for your efforts are great reminders that you are doing well and are certainly to be celebrated. Never turn away from a "thank you." Accept them graciously, and hold them in your heart. But the moment you think that you are better than That which you are a channel of, you lose all worthiness of your accolades. Acknowledge the Divine, the source of our great works and of our inspirations, and you will continue to do great deeds. But inject your own variations and ideas into what comes naturally, and you'll be just as good as an inexperienced rider who has fallen from his horse. God doesn't need help in knowing what to do. God just needs a *channel* to do what needs to be done.

3. Don't ever ask what's in it for you. This isn't about you in the first place. Your gifts are for *them*, the people you serve. Sure, we all need to make a living. If you follow rules 1 and 2 well, you'll never have to ask.

Once you lose sight of the big picture, you lose everything. This isn't about gain or reward. It *is* about playing your *vital* role in the Universe's master plan. To not recognize this means that you missed the point of your purpose. When this happens, your ego wrongly believes that it's all about you and what you can gain. Even if you struggle in life, your struggle does serve a purpose. For as hard as that may seem to believe, keeping that in mind is what keeps your heart full and your sense of purpose alive. So, what really *is* in it for you anyway? It's the satisfaction of knowing that you play an integral part in something amazing, even if your part seems small and insignificant or even painful in some way.

The "big picture" has to do with the Divine manifesting in this world as many people playing many roles. This includes as *you*. There will always be people who are poor or ill, and there will always be people who are there to help them in some way. Every restaurant has its owner and its dish washer. Every city has its mayor and its street sweeper. Without one, the other would have no purpose. In the same way, without *you*, the people that you come in contact with would not experience their life the way they do with you in it. They would not learn the same things, have the same experiences, or be in the same place in life. It is *necessary* for you to be there. It is paramount that you exist. In the end, it's not so much the role you played as it is the fact that you recognize that you are the Divine having manifested to play such a role.

4. Do not give of yourself for free just to attract customers. Those who do not contribute to their own healing process will remain in pain anyway.

There are many self-proclaimed "spiritual" natural health practitioners out there who believe that they should not charge for what they do, particularly energy healers. These are the very people that fail to recognize the value in what they do. Everything has a value, and for you to merely give something away validates that you see no worth in it. These people also fail to recognize how exactly energy healing works. Energy needs to be *exchanged* in order for healing to work. The practitioner must be willing to *accept* payment of some sort for his or her work in order to acknowledge the importance of the exchange. As for the receiver to not offer something in return, whether in monetary value or a bartered good or service, he or she does not place much value in the energy he or she is receiving, even if it is healing. Do not belittle what you do! It is a great work, and it needs the *reciprocating* movement of the divine energy in order to be of benefit.

5. Keep your struggles and your complaints away from your clients and especially away from your *prospective* clients. There is no reason why anyone should trust someone who oozes negative energy.

No one can build a viable business when they harbor negativity for very long. It is especially toxic for this negativity to be expressed to others. This is the main reason why I stopped associating myself with one of the business partners at U3: Body, Mind, & Spirit for some time. His "woe is me" laments over the fact that he has no clients of his own and his self-defeating belief that nobody takes him seriously made his energy quite repelling. Potential customers and associates were turned off by this, and they withdrew their interest in being involved with U3 because of this. These complaints were quite visible, taking place openly and on social media. When I called him on it, he turned against me. This is what happens when you feel you are a victim of circumstances instead of seeing everything, including your hardships, as forward progress.

Even if people don't actually see the self-immolation going on, they can certainly *feel* it when they are around you. The energy is like a cloud that hovers over you. Whether or not your own personal situation seems bad, you absolutely *must* create a warm, loving, healing environment for those that you serve if you want to build a business. This happens automatically when you get your ego out of the way. There is no negativity when the ego is silent. People will naturally be turned off by a person who exudes negative energy. Likewise, they will be naturally attracted to someone who radiates positive energy. I talk more about how this actually works in the chapter "Connections."

6. Open yourself up to the possibility that what you *think* you were meant to do in life is really not what the Universe wants you to do. Investigate the possibility that your calling is actually something you've never considered before. Your greatest success may, in fact, lie there.

When our career brings us plenty of satisfaction and monetary stability, we have no reason to question whether or not we are doing the right thing. But when things don't work out and we end up in an impoverished or unfulfilled state, even though we really wanted to do what we're doing, it's time to consider the possibility of another path. Maybe we invested a lot of time, effort, and money into it. To see all that go down the tubes is indeed disheartening. It doesn't mean you merely give up on your dreams. It means you contemplate that the Universe may have actually intended for you to do something else. Maybe you were destined to have a different role entirely in the big picture, something that may actually bring you greater abundance without much effort. Considering this possibility is always a better option than continuing to beat your head against a wall. Accepting this possibility will set the energy in motion toward the revelation of your true calling. After all, it is ego that causes you to cling to thoughts. In contrast, it is divine inspiration that leads you to freedom from the expectations of your thoughts.

7. Don't ever take a negative response personally. While the person you may be reaching out to obviously needs what you have to offer, only the lucky ones get to experience your gift. Treasure those people, and shake the rest off like sand from the bottom of your sandals. (Flat out ignoring you does count as a negative response.)

When you are in business for yourself, it is important to keep in mind that rejection comes with the territory. It is so common that books have been written just on how to handle it. Let's face it. Whether or not you like sales, if you let people know about what you have to offer and how you can help them, you *are* selling! The type of rejection that is so hard to take is when you get a negative, and sometimes arrogant, reaction from someone who is obviously in need of exactly what it is you are offering. In addition to such replies, receiving no response at all counts as a brush-off. Silence is not only a passive form of rejection but also a downright insult whereby the person is affirming that you are neither credible nor able to help him in his mind. It makes it all the sweeter when somebody *does* become a client and is grateful for what you do. It became easier for me to handle rejection by keeping in mind the miracles I've been a part of along the way as a healer and by knowing that only those who are *ready* to heal will ever be fortunate enough to experience what I do.

8. The truth will prevail in the hearts of others, your intended audience. Just keep putting your message out there, and those with whom it resonates will embrace it and follow through.

Your words and your blessings are not meant for everyone. Not all people can be so enlightened to the depth and importance of your message. Some people cannot comprehend your truth because they have different beliefs. It is not your job to convert people. It *is* your job to bring the birds of a feather together. If you have an utmost degree of confidence in what you stand for, then you are impermeable to the sticks and stones of the naysayers and the closed-minded. If you are true to your path, you will eventually find others who are true as well. Just keep doing what you're doing, and to thine own self be true.

It is true that the honest person oftentimes is the last to succeed professionally.[4] As an autie and an INFJ, I know this all too well. I never had much of a practice to speak of, and being a stone's throw from homelessness has been my reality all along. In fact, one of the best chiropractors ever to work on me was also very honest, soft spoken and lighthearted. He never had a big practice until two decades after he started when he bought the practice of his preceptor who had passed away. We aren't interested in bloated numbers to pad our egos and incomes. We have a message for a few chosen ears, for those interested in living better lives. Our message is not intended for people who merely want to relieve their pain. The successful servant will not compromise his integrity in order to meet a quota. He will stand true to a principle that the right people will follow.

It is not about shouting loudly to bring self-righteousness for a cause or ire to a foe. It is about strengthening a platform upon which those who abide by a certain truth can stand. There is strength in numbers, certainly. One never knows how many words it will take for the collective conscience to finally change. As the saying goes, rivers do not carve through rock primarily because of their force but because of their persistence. The purpose of your persistence is not to change people, although that may happen at times. Instead, it is to help the collective conscience grow in number and in surety, steadfastness, and conviction. In this way, the truth will prevail. It is destined to. Truth always wins in the end.

Obviously, these eight rules do not pertain to specific skills or techniques for selling or for building a clientele, or even to how you should do what you do. They are meant to be tenets upon which your frame of mind must be based in order to become largely successful. On the topic of entrepreneurship, a person on the autism spectrum may be at their best when they are their own boss. This automatically takes away the impending frustration that comes with trying to fit in at a particular work place and with catering to rules that don't exactly work with the way they think and process information. Because of such challenges, entrepreneurs on the autism spectrum may very well need advocates and people who can do the marketing work for them. In this way, they can concentrate on their strength, their gift — their purpose.

5

The Issues

Shortly after Becky and I started living together, I made it a regular thing to listen to the local emergency scanner radio online. During all those years I was involved in the world of firefighting, Emergency Medical Services, and fire policing, a scanner always hung from my belt like an extra appendage. It was a vital part of my very being. Because of this, I became quite keen to the difference in the nature and types of calls that are common nowadays compared to what had been considered usual all those years ago. I'm speaking specifically about psychiatric emergencies, acts of violence, people going into cardiac arrest, and, saddest of all, pediatric emergencies involving children with chronic illnesses. Nowadays, they are an everyday occurrence and were rarely ever heard of back in the 80s and early 90s. So, why the change? Those who warned of dangers in popular environmental and health-related practices foresaw such a rise in the types of illnesses we see today. They knew that things could not continue the way they were going without there being repercussions eventually.

In 1979, a progressive medical doctor by the name of Robert Mendelsohn published the first of three books which detail common medical procedures that have becomes staples to one's practice primarily because of profit instead of necessity. If he were to publish his books nowadays, they would probably be much thicker. Although many of Dr.

Mendelsohn's ideas may seem extreme even to the holistic practitioner, there was much truth to the more complex issues he discussed. He pointed out those procedures which can be considered unnecessary, and even downright dangerous, even though they are preferred because of how lucrative they are or because they make things easier on the doctor. A great deal of what happens in the world of health care seems to place the desires of the provider well above the needs of the patient. This can be related to the provider's own ego fueled by their sense of entitlement, the amount of education they went through, or because of the authority they have. A lot can also be due to misconceptions that have been accepted as truths over the years, truths that only a heretic or a mad person would dare to challenge.

Another question we need to ask is why society is so oblivious to the changes within itself as it goes along with the status quo. In retrospect, one has to wonder if these soapboxes of the educated, as opposed to the authoritarians, have some merit to them. While I was still a student chiropractor, I came to realize all too well that they really do. I also came to realize that those who do not care about the issues of today's world, those who would rather follow the piper's every word blindly, are the ones activists label as "sheeple." Sheeple simply go along with what society, the news media, and those who wear the big pants say without question while barking furiously at those that do question and show concern. In relation to Autism Spectrum Disorder in particular, although we are still not 100% sure of what causes it, we *do* know some of the things that could trigger its onset. Those who are more educated and who know how to do their own research are more affirmed of the triggers. The sheeple, on the other hand, just move along with the herd that is being led over the cliff. There are several common woes that society, especially in the United States, faces in today's world. Let's take a look at some of the health-related issues.

VACCINATION

Most people are very well aware of the growing anti-vaccination movement which is being fueled by the fear that vaccines may be causing many of the chronic illnesses people suffer from these days, especially autism. In reality, opposition to vaccination is nothing new. It's been around for as long as vaccines themselves. In the United States, we can trace opposition to the practice of vaccination as far back as 1722, although back then people opposed vaccination entirely for religious reasons[5]. Today it's because educated consumers are getting tired of the rhetoric being pushed on them by medical practitioners and their literature. The number of people being injured by vaccines is growing, and more and more types of vaccines are being marketed concurrently to the worsening of society's health overall.

Seeing a myriad of articles ranking the U.S. dead last among developed nations in its healthiness only adds to the grimness, such as the January 10, 2013 article by Grace Rubenstein published in *The Atlantic* which ranks the U.S. 17th. These startling statistics should raise a big red flag, and they do among educated and informed parents who want to *protect* their children from harm. They know that there is such a thing as the Vaccine Adverse Event Reporting System and that the National Vaccine Injury Compensation Program has paid out over $2.6B in damages since its inception in 1989[6]. They know that vaccines contain thimerosal, aluminum, formaldehyde[7], and other known neurotoxins that when added up over time can certainly damage the development of the neurological system[8]. They know that when more people begin to simply say "no" to whatever may potentially bring harm, the conscience of the society as a whole can be changed.

In addition to the concern about toxicity, there are the issues of effectiveness and of effect on a child's immune system. Many recent outbreaks of supposedly vaccine-preventable diseases have occurred among fully vaccinated populations. Even after receiving the flu vaccine, people continue to get the flu. Educated parents realize that many childhood diseases are no longer prevalent these days due to improvements in living standards and to the development of antibiotics, not primarily due to vaccination[9]. Besides, the death rates from diseases which were commonplace all those years ago were well on the decline in the United States and in the U.K. much earlier than when the vaccines were ever introduced[10]. Knowing this has many educated parents feeling safer with naturally-acquired immunity instead of subjecting their child to the potential dangers imposed by vaccines. Providing a child with natural antibodies from breast milk and eliciting a natural response through exposure (hence the popularity of pox parties) are always the better choice among nature-cognizant parents.

In addition to all the debate about metal adjuvants, adverse reactions, and how immunity is acquired, there exists a big issue with a little name: SV40. SV40 is an inherent virus found in Rhesus monkey kidney tissue, the main medium upon which antigens were cultivated decades ago, particularly for the polio vaccine. Even though it was discovered in 1961, and a federal law was written mandating that no vaccine should contain the virus, already-existing vaccines containing SV40 continued to be distributed supposedly right up until the late 1990s[11]. So, how does this affect humans? In 1992, DNA segments from the SV40 virus were showing up in human tumors[12]. And if that isn't scary enough, nowadays many antigens are grown on human diploid cells, i.e. aborted fetal tissue, instead. A study published in the September 2014 issue of the *Journal of Public Health and Epidemiology* shows that there is a direct correlation between the introduction of the use of aborted fetal tissue as a medium and a rise in the rate of autism[13].

And then there are some rather ridiculous beliefs that are better fodder for a science fiction novel than determining how an entire society should believe, such as the concepts of "herd immunity" and vaccinated children catching diseases from the unvaccinated. Herd immunity can never happen as a result of vaccination. It is a process only possible through naturally-acquired immunity. And when the vaccinated become sick from the very thing they were vaccinated against, the best example being the flu, it all gets chalked up to a "bad batch" of the vaccine or an aberrant strain. It could even be blamed on one having come in contact with an unvaccinated person. How these things might even work cannot be explained scientifically. Such fables abound in the mindset of the sheeple who are constantly being fed this foolishness by the very doctors that people depend on for the truth. These are excellent examples of fear-mongering at its best. I will talk more in-depth about vaccination in the chapter "What the Studies Show About Vaccination."

PRESCRIPTION MEDICATIONS

Most people believe that medications are placed on the market only after they've been proven by the Food and Drug Administration (FDA) to be safe and effective. In reality, this is not at all the way it works. According to Larry Chiaramonte, MD, coauthor of *Asthma Allergies Children: A Parent's Guide,* there are three phases to an FDA trial. In phase one, you have to prove that the drug is not lethal. Phase two must prove it is effective for the indicated condition. In phase three, you pay doctors to administer it to 5,000 - 10,000 patients to ascertain wider effectiveness and examine for side effects. After phase three, if the benefits outweigh complications and side effects caused by the drug by a convincing degree, you can put it on the market. But that's not all there is to it. Even after phase three, a drug must prove itself. Complications and side effects that never showed up in clinical trials will eventually show up in practice.

During all phases, the medications, though still experimental, are actually prescribed to patients. It's all trial and error from there. What is most disturbing about all this is how the third phase is conducted. The FDA relies on data that *sponsors* submit when deciding on whether a drug should be approved[14]. The FDA is not the one studying the drug, and the sponsor, i.e. the pharmaceutical company, has ample funds available to pay the ones prescribing the drugs to paint a pretty picture. This is quite the example of callous disregard for a person's health when profits are more important. The organization ProCon.org, a nonprofit organization that discusses the pros and cons of controversial issues, lists 35 medications which have been pulled from the market because of their dangers, some which had been in use for decades.

Let's face it, prescription drugs are the 4th leading cause of death in the U.S. *when properly prescribed*[15]. Yes, during the twelve years I was part of mainstream medicine, I've certainly seen many lives being saved by medications when administered properly, including my own. But I also saw, firsthand, the damage that medications can do. One such example was when I was given a dose of Demerol which was intended for the person in the next hospital room. I spent the next eighteen hours in and out of consciousness. Another example is the high number of middle-aged men who suddenly develop muscle weakness and pain in their legs after being prescribed a statin drug. (I talk more about statin drugs later in this chapter.) Whether they are experimental and not yet approved by the FDA or have been on the market for a long time, medications are just plain dangerous. Another common disaster, especially with the elderly, is that medications are often prescribed in conjunction with conflicting drugs which when combined could have deadly results. I've seen this time and time again during all those years I worked as an Emergency Medical Technician. Oftentimes, the prescribing physicians may not even know of these dangers.

I am particularly disturbed when I see people being prescribed psychotropic drugs for medical conditions that the physician would rather not investigate further such as fibromyalgia, Chronic Fatigue Syndrome, Lyme Disease, and similar autoimmune disorders. Without considering any other possible diagnosis, sufferers of such conditions are quickly dismissed with scrip in hand for medications such as Prozac, Effexor, and Xanax. Personally, I consider this malpractice. In a paper which was presented at the press conference sponsored by the Alliance for Human Research Protection (AHRP) at the FDA Public Hearing on Antidepressants and Suicide held on September 14, 2004, Dr. Peter Breggin, author and expert in psychiatry, points out not only the prevalence of violent behavior, particularly in children, resulting from the use of common antidepressants but also how the dangers of such medications have been hidden from the public. Much of this coverup was a joint effort between Eli Lily, manufacturer of Prozac, and the FDA. Naturally, there would be no financial benefit for the FDA to go against its biggest monetary supporters!

In addition to the issues of prescription medications being inherently dangerous and their manufacturers and sponsors paying out big bucks to get them approved regardless, there are other safety factors that need to be looked at. Once the medications are in the hands of the consumers, other problems may arise. Is the intended patient taking the right dosage for his or her condition? Does the patient take the medication regularly and in the right way? Do the drugs have the chance of falling into the wrong hands? This is of particular concern among youngsters since prescription drugs, including cough and cold medications, are the most commonly abused substances, next to marijuana and alcohol, among Americans age 14 and older[16]. Painkillers are sought for their opioid properties, Valium and Xanax for their calming effects, and Ritalin and Adderall, which are used to treat ADHD, for their stimulant effects. All of these issues are the very reasons why medications should be used sparingly and only when necessary. In fact, as I see it, medication is necessary to stabilize the condition of a person who is in a crisis situation and *only until* a viable non-pharmaceutical treatment option can be found for maintenance care. Hence, relying on alternative medicine and holistic healing as a first line of treatment is a rapidly-growing trend among the educated population.

So, how then is a *consumer* to know if a medication they've been prescribed is safe? This is not information you can depend on your primary care provider to divulge. It just doesn't work that way. One thing you could do is buy a Physicians Desk Reference, which is an annual encyclopedia of every prescription drug on the market today. Every single drug has a list of potential side effects associated with it. But the more accurate source one can turn to is the FDA's Center for Drug Evaluation and Research. This organization created the Drug Safety Communications program, which is geared mainly toward consumers, to advise of impending risks of FDA-approved drugs (obviously ones that had already passed through the initial three-phased study period). Their advisories are then published on the FDA's website.

CHILDBIRTH IN THE U.S.

Let's take a look at the way most children are born in the United States. Both the high rate of cesarean births and mothers being placed in the typical lithotomy position during delivery present risks that can easily be avoided. The proven safer methods that one can opt for are vaginal birth in a squatting or a side-lying position. A research article published in the Journal of Perinatal Education suggests six Healthy Birth Practices that paint a picture of what is ideal in a holistic model, many of which are practiced in most privately-owned birthing centers[17]. The same article mentions that much of what is common practice in the medical setting is not evidence-based and can lead to unexpected complications. In March 2010, I produced a half-hour video in which I detailed the biomechanics and effects of birth trauma which often results from typical birth practices such as the use of extraction devices and forced deliveries. In my video, I cite Abraham Towbin, M.D., a Harvard-educated neuropathologist, whose studies proved that the force placed on the baby's head can cause direct damage and impairment to the undeveloped nervous system. There is much to be discussed regarding this topic alone, and I will go further into detail regarding the direct effects of birth trauma on the nervous system later in this book.

One viable alternative to traditional childbirth is the growing trend of underwater birthing. In an article written by Barbara Harper, RN, published in the Summer 2014 edition of the Journal of Perinatal Education, Harper indicates that many prominent hospitals around the world offer this safe and much more comforting option. Although underwater birthing is practiced widely around the world, its popularity in the U.S. is only now starting to catch on. Harper also discusses many international studies which point out that there were no complications due to respiratory compromise, development of fetal infection, perineal trauma, or hypothermia, and that there was far less need for any medical intervention due to labor pains. There was, however, objection to the whole practice of underwater birthing from both the American Academy of Pediatrics and the American College of Obstetricians and Gynecologists (notice they are both "American") who both touted loudly the usual fear-mongering nonsense.

THE HIGH-CHOLESTEROL MYTH

There is a long-standing myth that high cholesterol is a bad thing. Two days after I had open heart surgery, an aortic valve replacement which saved my life, the surgeon made a follow-up visit to my bedside. One rather surprising thing he said to me sticks in my head to this day. He said, point blank, "Over the years you'll hear your cardiologists telling you that you need to lower your cholesterol. Don't pay any attention to it because it's all hogwash." I was nineteen years old at the time, and I had no idea of some of the medical mayhem that existed in health care back then. This shed light on the games being played by the medical profession before I was ever even involved in it. Fast forward almost thirteen-and-a-half years to the time I was a student chiropractor. On one particular day, while studying a particular cadaver in the human dissection lab, I was told that the person had passed on from Coronary Artery Disease. As I opened the left coronary artery, a rather large blockage was evident. I noticed, however, that it was not caused by a buildup of plaque or cholesterol. It was from triglycerides. That brought to mind the words of the cardiologist who had cared for me when I lived in Valparaiso, Indiana three years earlier: "Don't worry about your cholesterol numbers. It's the triglycerides you have to keep an eye on."

Apparently, very few cardiologists and primary care providers bother to tell people the truth. It's much more profitable for them to write a prescription for a medication to lower cholesterol. Albeit, some physicians believe that what they were taught is indeed factual and that they are doing the right thing. Over the years that I've been in practice, I've had several middle-aged to elderly male patients come to me with unexplained severe "nerve" pain in their legs, including my own dad. My first question to them is regarding whether or not they are taking a statin drug. Statins are the most common type of prescription cholesterol-lowering medication. Almost always, the answer is "yes." An article published by the Mayo Clinic lists this type of pain as a side effect, among other "rare" (according to them) problems including liver damage[18]. A friend of mine in Minnesota died of cardiac arrest only days after commencing usage of a statin drug. Despite the known dangers and potentially deadly and commonly debilitating effects, statin drugs continue to be pushed in order to correct a mythical disease known as "hypercholesterolemia," or high cholesterol. But why?

The whole high-cholesterol-causes-heart-disease myth began when Nikolai N. Anichkov, a Russian-born German researcher of unknown professional background (other than that he was a student at the Imperial Military Medical Academy in St. Petersburg, Russia) did an experiment where he measured the effects of "foreign bodies" on the cardiac tissue of rabbits. When cholesterol was introduced into the tissues, the cell structure changed, and the tissue lost its contractibility. This study was concluded in 1913, and it paved the way for other studies into the cause and physiology of atherosclerosis[19]. Recent discussions, however, bring up points of fallacy in Anichkov's study since it didn't involve an actual diet being fed to the rabbits. Some articles even note that the Anichkov study was not reproducible in other types of animals or when certain physiological factors were changed, such as thyroid function.

The big push toward creating a high-cholesterol scare in order to market cholesterol lowering drugs came soon after the Framingham Heart Study began in 1948. This study set out to identify common factors in the development of cardiovascular disease. Even though several other studies debunked the link between cholesterol and cardiovascular disease[20], the Framingham study, which continues to this day, remains the golden standard by which the medical profession determines its treatment options. Even though the Framingham study itself hasn't found any direct link between diet and cholesterol level[21], the medical establishment prefers to believe in such a fable. It makes for a great way to scare people into compliance.

Despite the fact that there was no evidence to definitively prove that diet and cholesterol levels are related, and despite the fact that cholesterol is *naturally produced* by the liver, the search was on to create a cholesterol-lowering drug. In 1971, a Japanese biochemist named Akira Endo developed a drug named Mevastatin. Although it was never widely distributed because of its adverse effects, Merck & Co., Inc. picked up the idea in 1975 and developed it into something marketable[22], "marketable" meaning that it was easy to capitalize on the supposed data suggesting that cholesterol has something to do with cardiovascular disease. Thus, we have a multi-billion-dollar industry based on a belief, a belief that is being fed to people in the U.S. as truth thereby enforcing the "need" of such a drug. Despite the studies proving the dangers of statin drugs, the belief that cholesterol causes heart disease coupled with the fact that statins can lower LDL, the supposed "bad" cholesterol, the promoting and prescribing of these drugs is kept alive. One such study that proves the dangers of statin drugs was done by Harumi Okuyama et al. and was published in the February 6, 2015 issue of *Expert Review of Clinical Pharmacology*. It showed that statin drugs actually *cause* atherosclerosis and congestive heart failure

THE "COCONUT OIL IS BAD FOR YOU" MYTH

In accordance with the previous topic, there are people who are expert in the fabled clogged-pipes-due-to-diet theory of where heart and vascular diseases come from. They promulgate the scientifically-debunked scare that eating saturated fats can cause such illnesses. While it is true that fats, proteins, and carbohydrates all need to constitute a balanced percentage of the daily diet, it is grossly unfair to say that any one of them is at fault when it comes to the development of a particular illness. As for saturated fat specifically, the scare comes from the idea that eating them raises cholesterol levels in the body. Since coconut oil is high in saturated fat (yet not at the top of the list), it has ended up getting the bum rap. But when you realize that cholesterol is, first of all, actually regulated by the liver and, secondly, a major constituent of body cell structures, you can conclude that cholesterol itself isn't bad at all. One of the biggest studies proving that saturated fat has nothing to do with the development of either coronary heart disease (CHD) or cardiovascular disease (CVD) was published in 2010 with almost 350,000 subjects being examined for a diet-CHD/CVD link. Although 11,000 of the subjects had suffered CHD, CVD, or a stroke between 5 and 23 years after their initial intake examination, none of their conditions were related to the intake of saturated fats.[23]

The usage and availability of coconut oil have grown significantly in the past decade, largely due to a more health-conscious population promoting its benefits. It is evident when you can find various brands of coconut oil on supermarket shelves whereas years ago it was available only in health food stores. One would have to wonder, then, why coconut oil has suddenly come under attack even though there are other oils that contain a higher amount of saturated fat. Some food products have a greater amount of saturated fats in them than others with palm kernel oil, coconut oil, and butter having the highest in that order.[24] When you realize that several articles list some of the many benefits of coconut oil being fat-burning, antibacterial, appetite-reducing, mental clarity, cosmetic repairing, and even health maintaining for those who make coconut a staple in their diet, the reasons why more health care professionals are not singing its praises are dismaying. When you can help someone live a healthy lifestyle and improve their conditions using natural foods and remedies which they can concoct at home, what need is there for prescription medication?

I just talked about a few of my most notable grinds. There are many other examples of how the medical establishment makes billions in profit by feeding non-truths to people. In 1993, while working as a Respiratory Therapist at the Porter Memorial Hospital in Valparaiso, Indiana, I became quite a critic toward certain procedures I viewed as unnecessary. Two such examples are Intermittent Positive Pressure Breathing (IPPB) and the use of oxygen tents. While I was seen as an antagonist back in those days, it is evident that I was onto something since these two therapies, among others I was outspoken about, no longer exist.

THE DIAGNOSTIC CRITERIA OF DISEASES

Most people may be quite surprised to learn that diseases, both physical and mental, come and go simply by changing their diagnostic criteria. It happens *all* the time. For physical disorders, the criteria for evaluation and proper diagnostic testing are determined by the associations who oversee the management of the disorder. For example, The Expert Committee on the Diagnosis and Classification of Diabetes Mellitus decides how the various types of diabetes mellitus should be tested for and treated as well as what the signs and symptoms of the various forms are. Another example is the American College of Rheumatology, which determines the diagnostic criteria and treatment of rheumatoid arthritis and other rheumatic diseases. Sometimes, diagnostic criteria for a disease can vary from one country to another. A good example of this is with Sjögren's Syndrome, whereby both the American College of Rheumatology and the American-European Consensus Group had their own differing standards. Mental illnesses are handled differently. Diagnostic criteria are determined and updated regularly by the American Psychiatric Association. The new standards are then published in the next edition of the Diagnostic and Statistical Manual of Mental Disorders, or DSM for short.

Now that we know this, we can clearly see how certain diseases and disorders came to be and how some were eliminated. Did you know that homosexuality was once considered a mental disorder? That is until, in 1973, the American Psychiatric Association simply took a vote and decided it was time to no longer list it as a disorder. The vote was largely due to changes in societal norms[25]. And what really *did* happen to polio? In 1996, polio merely slipped under the umbrella of Acute Flaccid Paralysis (AFP) which includes many other paralytic conditions such as Guillain-Barre Syndrome (for which I had treated people during my days as a Respiratory Therapist), Transverse Myelitis, and Chinese Paralytic Syndrome[26]. But the decline in polio began in the "immediate pre-vaccine era" due to improvements that were made in the sanitation systems in the U.S. Thus, we have the eradication of polio, highly hailed to the vaccine. In that light, the purpose of the polio vaccine was, therefore, *not* to wipe out the disease but to increase immunity against it now that people were no longer subject to its primary source, contaminated water.[27] For another example, let's take a look at how most cases of autism came to be — merely by changing the diagnostic criteria and listing it as a spectrum disorder in the DSM-IV-TR[28]. By doing so, we included on the spectrum 59% of the people tested using the DSM-III guidelines who had been deemed to not have autism[29].

And there you have it. Want to cure a disease? Change the way it's diagnosed. Want to create one? Throw together a group of signs and symptoms and invent some sort of "abnormal" lab test result to diagnose it. That's *precisely* what happens to create a multi-billion-dollar scare! This is called "disease mongering,"[30] and it happens more often than you realize. It is *exactly* how high cholesterol came to be a treatable disease and is also how "metabolic syndrome" was invented[31]. But the truth is that not all the blame lies with the organization that created the disease or the pharmaceutical company that manufactures its cure. It also lies with the medical practitioner who is willing to put his hands in the money pot and diagnose the "illness"[32]. In retrospect, should we really be making gods out of the men and women who wear the white coats? Unfortunately, it is the people who never question their motives and methods who keep them in power. As for those who know better, we will seek the safer alternative, educate ourselves, and question *everything*.

There are many other ways in which people are being duped, such as Monsanto trying to assure that genetically modified organisms are safe and fit for human consumption, dentists telling patients that there is no harm in amalgam tooth fillings, municipal water authorities continuing to put fluoride in their water despite the outcries and evidence against it, and the dairy industry's claim that raw milk is harmful. Discussion on these topics would fill an entire book, and this book is concerned with what is going on in health care today. Thanks to the growing number of educated minds, people are awakening to the need to do their own research and are creating activist movements and organizations opposed to such harmful practices. Changes are being made, slowly but surely. Yet, unless the people who initiate the harmful practices and policies suddenly develop a moral conscience, these diseases and adversities will only continue.

6

Autism: Causes & Cures

Whenever I hear people mention the need to "cure" people with autism, I can't help but think that these people have no idea about the brilliance that many people with autism are endowed with. Maybe they are the parents or caretakers of children or adults on the lower end of the functioning spectrum? Maybe they heard too much rhetoric from a well-known autism-related organization that describes everyone with autism as being a burden (the same organization which those who know better adamantly boycott)? Maybe they know a person with autism who suffers from one or more concomitant, or associated, conditions? In any case, it is important to keep in mind that autism cannot be cured. One *might*, however, experience significant improvement in their physical ailments or mental function by trying a certain diet or therapy. The thing is that there are so many certain diets and therapies out there that it is difficult for a person to know where to start. The most important point to keep in mind is that when you find something that helped you, you found something that helped probably just you and a given percentage of other people. You did *not* find a cure-all, and such a find should never be touted as such. To do so could lead to much frustration for many who try *your* "proven" method.

Speaking of concomitant conditions, one disorder I find to be of great intrigue is, collectively, digestive problems. It seems we in the health and scientific communities are missing something obvious. This is not to say there aren't other factors in the development or treatment of autism symptoms. It is to say that there is an elephant in the room that is invisible to most. Before I go further into detail about this particular topic, I will point out some apparent facts that seem to get lost in the shuffle of all the bits of info being pored through by inquiring minds:

- During neurological development, children with Autism Spectrum Disorder (ASD) can form extra nerve synapses in the brain which lead to alterations in the way certain areas of the brain function[33].

- There is a direct and significant relationship between children receiving the MMR vaccine before their third birthday and the onset of autism[34].

- There is significant evidence of a direct correlation between in-utero exposure to neurotoxins, such as pesticides and teratogens, and the development of disorders such as autism, intellectual disabilities, and even developmental abnormalities of the reproductive organs[35].

- Several problems that crop up during labor and shortly after birth appear to increase a child's risk of developing autism. Birth trauma increases one's risk of developing autism fivefold. A low oxygen level during delivery, especially during difficult or high-risk deliveries, and growth retardation are very good predictors of the development of autism. Recent studies place the favorability of these findings well ahead of the old theory that autism is a genetic disorder[36]. Some theories suggest that this low oxygen level is due to clamping of the umbilical cord before the cord stops pulsating, thereby reducing the amount of oxygenated blood the newborn may benefit from.

- In October 2014, it was reported that over 100 genetic mutations have been implicated in the development of autism. These mutations were found mainly in genes involved in making protein, and several more are expected to be discovered as a greater part of the human genome is studied. The mutations occur "spontaneously," and they are implicated in at least 30% of all cases of autism. These are not hereditary in nature, and the mutations are reported to occur during embryonic development[37]. Perhaps the most notable of these mutations is to the methylenetetrahydrofolate reductase (NAD(P)H), or MTHFR, gene. MTHFR is an enzyme that plays a vital role in the production of amino acids and folate.

As you can see, there are scientifically-validated arguments for whichever "cause" you choose to stand by and fight against. It could very well be that if you put three people with autism together, each one may have had a different cause of their autism. One may have had a vaccine reaction while another one suffered from a low oxygen level at birth. The third person may have had a traumatic event that impaired his neurological development, such as a life-threatening illness in infancy. The lattermost situation describes me personally. However, that's not to say that the salmonella illness that nearly killed me at the age of five months was what cause me to have autism, although it is the best guess. It could also be that my weakened immune state made me more susceptible to adverse vaccine reactions. This is also why one cannot responsibly say that if they found something which helped them or their child with their autism symptoms or with a concomitant condition that that something will certainly help somebody else.

One thing I know for sure is that there is a high prevalence of digestive disorders among people with ASD. I've seen a lot of this in fellow auties I came to know at the autism support groups I attended over the years. Even Temple Grandin made yogurt a staple in her daily diet when she had attacks of colitis. Many natural health activists might point the finger at gluten in the diet causing the autism, but this argument is easily debunked by the results of a study done on this very topic which was published in the May 2013 issue of *Clinical Therapeutics*. This study shows that even though a variety of symptoms may be present in those with gluten sensitivity, no evidence had been noted in the improvement of autism symptoms after switching to a gluten-free diet[38]. On the other hand, there is growing evidence of a link between intestinal hyperpermeability, or Leaky Gut Syndrome, and autism[39].

Along the same line of thought, in Dr. Andrew Wakefield's retracted study that had been published in *The Lancet* in which he links the onset of behavioral symptoms to the timing of his subjects having received the MMR vaccine, he identified that every one of his subjects suffered from some kind of intestinal illness. Although his study consisted of a very small study group, I really think he was on to something. In an article published in *The Atlantic* on June 10, 2013, Dr. Kara Margolis, a pediatric gastroenterologist at New York Presbyterian Hospital and a researcher at

Columbia University Medical Center, points out that behaviors not typical in autism, such as aggression and self-harm, which in themselves are highly prevalent in people with autism, may, in fact, stem from gastrointestinal issues. She points out that once the underlying gut issues are treated, the adverse behaviors can be reversed. She also points out that since 90% of all the serotonin in the body is found in the gut, such issues are typically reversed by placing focus on treating the serotonin imbalance in the gut as opposed to labeling and treating a digestive disorder per se.

Intestinal problems and autism seem to go hand in hand. But why? Although there have been numerous medically-based studies and conjectures regarding theoretical causes with no real conclusions, several reports regarding the presence of toxins such as glyphosate in wheat products, breast milk, and even in vaccines themselves are coming to light. These reports are being made by people with no connection to any pharmaceutical companies or makers of herbicides or pesticides. If ties did exist, it is quite certain that such data would not be made public, just as the CDC intentionally hid data proving that the onset of debilitating forms of autism had a much higher rate of occurring immediately following administration of the MMR vaccine[40].

Glyphosate is an herbicide (weed killer) that is commonly sprayed on genetically modified crops just before they are harvested. It functions by disrupting the protein-assimilating pathways of its target plants. A study done by Anthony Samsel and Stephanie Seneff showed that the likelihood of glyphosate doing the same to vital metabolic pathways in humans was clearly defined[41]. This includes damaging the health of beneficial microbes found in the human gut. In another study done by Zen Honeycutt and

Stephanie Seneff, the presence of glyphosate in breast milk was detected even when the study's subjects intentionally avoided genetically modified products[42]. In yet another study done by Honeycutt and Seneff, glyphosate was found to be present in several vaccines, particularly the MMR II vaccine[43]. In the same study, Seneff suggests that glyphosate made its way into the vaccines because the medium upon which the antigens are grown are of animal origin, and the animals from which the media came were fed GMO products which were treated with the herbicide.

All in all, I give the best credibility to the research done by Dr. Abraham Towbin on birth trauma and its debilitating effects on neurological development. Dr. Towbin studied more than 2,000 infants who had died from SIDS. He found that a typical obstetric birth can traumatize the neck of the newborn leading to brain and spinal cord injury and could even result in death[44]. Dr. Towbin puts a lot of the blame on extraction devices used during C-section deliveries. Another study done on birth trauma done in Denmark in 2014 by Hans Bisgaard, M.D. showed that children born by C-section have a higher rate of various disorders including inflammatory bowel disease[45].

What does birth trauma have to do with digestive disorders? This can be explained with basic anatomy and physiology. There are two particular nerves that originate within the brain and exit through the base of the skull, the right and left Vagus nerves. As they wander down through the neck, the chest, and on to the abdomen, they send branches to various parts of the body. These nerves, as well as every nerve in the body, are the communication links between the various parts of the body and the brain. In the neck, the Vagus nerves pass in close proximity to the front of the very top vertebra in the neck, the "Atlas." Mechanical injury during the birth process, and also head and neck injuries later in life, may cause the Atlas to shift out of alignment, or subluxate. Depending on which direction the Atlas shifts, it can place direct pressure on either of the Vagus nerves. Placing even a slight amount of pressure on *any* nerve is enough to disrupt the normal function of that nerve thereby altering the normal flow of communication between the body part or parts which that nerve goes to and the brain. Because the Vagus nerves terminate along the digestive tract, an Atlas misalignment can, and often does, cause disruption of the function of the digestive tract.

Now that we looked at just some of the potential causes of autism, we can talk about "cures." As stated before, contrary to what some self-promoting people who claim to have had success with one thing or another say, autism cannot be cured. Unless you can come up with a Whovian procedure to reverse the overgrowth of nerve synapses in the brain once they have occurred or a magical way to make a person on the autism spectrum suddenly start acting *and thinking* according to *your* expectations, I would never mention the word "cure." In fact, the remainder of this chapter will focus on practices designed to help the person with autism integrate with and function in the world around him.

First, I will talk about the controversial yet overly-popular Applied Behavior Analysis therapy, or ABA. Yes controversial, especially among the auties, and yes overly-popular, as it is practiced in most schools that have autism programs. This is mostly due to the fact that it is just about the only program paid for by most insurance companies including state funds. In a nutshell, the gist of ABA is to "train away" unwanted behaviors. Without a rhyme or reason as to why they are being treated as such, many children with ASD think they are being disciplined. This leads to much frustration and the feeling that they aren't "good enough." All you have to do is search for "ABA dangers" online to read story upon story about how ABA can traumatize children. It is a long and grueling program which most children do not have the attention span for. Adults with ASD whom I know personally that went through ABA when they were children all had one thing to say: "It felt horrible to be trained to be a robot." Many letters have appeared on autism-related websites from parents whose children suffered from Post-Traumatic Stress Disorder shortly after beginning the ABA program. Although there may be ABA therapists and parents out there who will argue that having their child go through ABA therapy has been nothing short of successful, I would rather hear it from the autie him/herself. They are, after all, people with feelings and not mindless robots.

Enter newer behavioral programs, ones which teach the parents to *connect* with their child in order to find out *why* the child is displaying a certain behavior. When there is understanding, unwanted and inappropriate behaviors can be changed or eliminated by helping the child to develop a new way of thinking. Now you have a synergy, a win-win situation, which benefits both the child and the parent. The best example I can bring up is the Son-Rise Program, which was voted the #1 autism therapy at the 2011 AutismOne conference. Yet, for how effective the program is with helping the parent and child form a viable communication bond, it has its share of drawbacks. The parent or teacher needs to travel to Sheffield, Massachusetts for five days of training. The startup program costs $2,200, although financial aid and scholarships are available. Also, former employees of The Option Institute, the organization owned by the founders of the program, have some rather negative comments regarding its business practices. Lastly, after having spoken with a program representative myself, I came to learn that they tout the program as an autism "cure," a huge red flag in my book.

Since the requirements of the Son-Rise program may not be so feasible for most, the question becomes one of finding a program that is suitable for someone who doesn't have the time to travel or the money to put into it. Unfortunately, it is difficult for any single recommendation to be made since there are many different types of behavioral modification therapies. In my research, I counted at least seventeen different named therapies or programs. Perhaps a good place to start is with a popular therapy called Floortime. Whether you like the Developmental, Individual-differences, Relationship-based (DIR) model or the Greenspan Floortime Model, the goal is to establish communication through connection and focusing on the building blocks of healthy development rather than on discipline and training. Ultimately, one must research the various programs and choose what they feel is best for them.

For adults on the spectrum, there is a program called Problem Solving Therapy (PST). This program is specifically designed to help adults cope with stressful situations. It has been proven effective in helping people who suffer from deep depression as well. PST offers a seven-step approach to dealing with a variety of life situations that the individual needs to cope with and work through. It entails a series of twelve sessions whereby the individual's ability to work his own way through his problems increases with each session. Numerous studies have shown PST to be more effective than both Supportive Therapy (ST) and Cognitive Behavioral

Therapy (CBT) in achieving the same goals. For adults on the spectrum in particular, PST may be most suitable due to the fact that people with autism have a more sensitive nature and due to their typical rulemaking approach to adapting to new situations.

In addition to behavior modification programs, there are plenty of treatments and therapies, both medical and alternative, which focus on keeping one's concomitant conditions and mental status in check. Medicine is used to keep symptoms under control, not as a means of curing anything. Dosages must be closely monitored due to the fact that people with ASD are very sensitive even to minute changes. As for the alternative medicine options such as chelation therapy or amino acid replacement therapy, it is assumed that the person's autism is due to the theoretical cause being treated. That's not to say they do not work. They indeed do work for a percentage of people. But they should never, as I stated before, be touted as a cure-all. Let's examine some of the medical and alternative medicine options.

Some of the most common disorders and adversities that exist alongside ASD are sleep problems, ADHD, meltdowns, and anxiety. Although concomitant conditions are not inherent to autism, they often arise due to either neurological development issues or because of difficulty with sensory, learning, or social processing and integration. These are all hallmark problems with autism. Usually, when medications are needed, the dosages are minuscule, oftentimes less than what a person without ASD would normally be prescribed. That's how reactive a person on the spectrum can be to even a trace amount of a medication. Typical medications prescribed are Ritalin or Adderall for ADHD, Ambien or Lunesta for sleep disorders, and Xanax or Ativan for anxiety. Another problem that can be encountered is depression for which Prozac, Paxil, or Zoloft are commonly prescribed. People on the lower-functioning end of the spectrum may have seizure disorders for which Depakote and Klonopin are the more commonly prescribed medications.

When dosed right and prescribed appropriately, these medications can certainly be a boon in helping a person with ASD function well. Even well-known speakers who have autism admit that without taking their minuscule doses of Prozac, they would never be able to get up in front of people to give presentations. The dangerous part is when something doesn't work for a person yet the same remedy is tried at a higher dose instead of switching to another medication altogether. For example, in cases of severe and unrelenting outbursts, the drug Haldol is the drug of choice for some medical providers. It is designed to bring fits of rage under control. It is also often prescribed to control the tics associated with Tourette's Disorder. I've seen this medication do wonders during my days as a private duty visiting nurse. But for as effective as it is for some, it does nothing for others. For the ones whose explosive episodes remain untouched by Haldol, perhaps Risperdal might do better. It's all a game of trials and errors, one which the medical establishment is often reluctant to play.

Because medical intervention is a game of chance, and a dangerous one at that due to all the medication side effects and high chances of error, many people feel safer turning to alternative medicine practices. Ever since 1990, more people in the general population have been visiting practitioners of alternative medicine on a whole, with chiropractors leading the statistics, than general practice MDs[46]. As far as alternative medicine goes, there are two schools of thought.

One promotes outside-in remedies such as herbal/vitamin supplementation and diet management to replace medical treatment. The inside-out approach, on the other hand, encourages the use of physical and mental exercises that promote and potentiate the body's own innate ability to heal. Such practices include chiropractic, first and foremost, Reiki, yoga, and meditation. Again, there are many different types of therapies, and to explain and enumerate them all would result in an entire encyclopedia. I discussed in detail how chiropractic and Reiki work in the chapter "The Book of Healing" in my book *The Doctor Is In*. Both are practices which I had used, and continue to use, with great success in helping people with ASD feel and function notably better, particularly when realigning a subluxated Atlas, which I will talk about in detail later in this book.

7

What the Studies Show About Vaccination

When I am presented with an article about health and medicine, I just have to wonder where the information came from sometimes. A well-researched article will have its references cited, yet many of the ones I come across do not. What gets me upset is when I write articles and people feel the information is bogus even when my references are clearly stated. This reaction usually comes from those who would rather not have their longstanding beliefs challenged or proven wrong. I've been in the health care field since August 11, 1982. I've seen the good, the bad, and the ugly of both mainstream and alternative medicine. I don't talk out of my hat like some self-proclaimed natural health activists do, or like staunch conformists to the medical mayhem for that matter. I never say something just to fit into a certain subculture or to make myself sound like an authority. Having a doctorate degree gives one a greater responsibility to state facts. Misleading people, especially when they are already part of the sheeple norm, is never a good idea. In this chapter, I list some actual studies that were published in peer-reviewed journals proving the points I and others often make about how dangerous the practice of vaccination is. Articles published in peer-reviewed journals are the golden standard by which all credible and accurate reporting is made.

Before I point out what the studies say, it is most important to keep in mind that there is no substitute for seeing the damages for yourself. During my internship, when I was still studying to become a Doctor of Chiropractic, I would often see vaccine-damaged children in our clinic. Their parents would bring them there in hopes of recovering some of the mental and physical capabilities they lost shortly after being vaccinated. That was in 1999. I never anticipated just how commonly-encountered and widespread vaccine-induced neurological defects would be. The current schedule of recommended childhood vaccines is far more comprehensive than those of generations ago. In 1983, only eleven vaccines were "required" before the age of sixteen. By 2016, that number grew to eighteen vaccines before the age of just six. Yet, no study has ever been done on the safety or the efficacy of such a schedule. There are plenty of studies, however, that show the evident dangers of it.

One such study was published in the February 2014 issue of *Journal of Molecular and Genetic Medicine*. This study, done by J. Barthelow Classen, M.D., shows clear evidence of "vaccine-induced immune overload" which leads to rapidly-increasing childhood epidemics such as Types I & II diabetes, metabolic disorders, inflammatory diseases, and even autism. In another study published in the Jan-Feb 1983 issue of *The Pediatric Infectious Diseases Journal*, it was proven that there is a high incidence of Sudden Infant Death Syndrome (SIDS) shortly after administration of the DTP vaccine (of which DTaP is a supposed "safer" version), though they list these occurrences as "temporal," or coincidental. Still another study published in the August 2016 issue of *Journal of Immunology Research* shows a high incidence of severe neurological symptoms including memory loss, fainting, depression, Chronic Fatigue Syndrome, insomnia, and many others within two months of receiving an HPV vaccine. Again, these occurrences were passed off as coincidental. The list goes on and on, and I found too many studies to count proving how dangerous and even deadly the practice of vaccination is.

So why, then, does it continue? Why are more and more "required" vaccines being added to the mess? Oddly enough, it has nothing to do with health care at all, nothing to do with the wellness and safety of your child. It is all about profitability. According to the *Global Human Vaccines Market 2016-2020*, the market for existing and upcoming vaccines is expected to generate $55B worldwide, with much of that growth credited to the HPV vaccine, and with most vaccines being given in the U.S. alone.[47] And because pharmaceutical companies are exempt from liability for injury and death caused by vaccines ever since the passing of the National Vaccine Injury Act in 1986, they have absolutely no incentive to make their vaccines any safer.[48] Even when mercury started being phased out as a vaccine adjuvant sometime after 1999 (in all except the annual flu vaccine), its replacement aluminum has proven to be just as toxic. Here are a few studies proving its harmful effects on humans:

- Petrovsky, Nikolai, Aguilar, Julio Cesar. "Vaccine adjuvants: Current state and future trends". *Immunology and Cell Biology*. Sept. 28, 2004. Vol. 82, Iss. 5, pp. 488-496. Nature Publishing Group. Web. Feb. 9, 2015.

This study compares adjuvants, or compounds added to vaccines to boost antigen effectiveness. Although aluminum-based compounds are the most common adjuvants used, they "rarely induce cellular immune responses." This article clearly lists neurotoxicity as a "limitation." Also noted in the article is that (my commentaries are in parentheses) "High aluminium (aluminum) levels in the body predominately affect the brain and bone tissues" and "Aluminium (aluminum) intoxication has also been associated with Amyotrophic Lateral Sclerosis (ALS, or Lou Gehrig's Disease) and Alzheimer's disease." Albeit, these conditions are most noted in people with impaired kidney function.

- Lee, Sing, Han. "Topological conformational changes of human papillomavirus (HPV) DNA bound to an insoluble aluminum salt—A study by low-temperature PCR". *Advances in Biological Chemistry*. Feb. 26, 2013. Vol. 3, No. 1, pp. 76-85. Scientific Research Publishing Inc. Web. Feb. 10, 2015

After the FDA first reported that there were no viral DNA components in the Gardasil vaccine, the above study proved otherwise. Dr. Lee found non-B-conformations, or the type of DNA that has been implicated in "approximately 20 neurological diseases, approximately 50 genomic disorders…, and several psychiatric diseases[49]." After being advised of this study's findings in September 2011 by SaneVax, Inc., a watchdog group promoting safe vaccine practices, the FDA revised its statement to read, "Based on the scientific information available to the FDA, Gardasil continues to be safe and effective, and its benefits continue to outweigh its risks[50]."

On that note, as I research countless articles regarding vaccination, I see two recurring statements, neither of which have been proven to be true: that vaccines have saved thousands of lives, and that serious complications are "rare." While I find these themes to be redundant at best, all the evidence shows otherwise, whether it be by case or coincidence. Articles that state percentages and populations that have been helped by vaccination do not cite where such statistics came from. I find no such studies having been done using any sort of study or control groups to prove such. In addition, no study has ever been funded by an independent group, that is one who is in no way associated with a drug manufacturer or medically-based organization. One thing is for certain, though, and that is that both mass vaccination and the increasing number of vaccines given are concurrent with the rise in illnesses such as diabetes, Multiple Sclerosis, Chronic Fatigue Syndrome, fibromyalgia, and with mental disorders such as depression and bipolar disorder. Let's look at a few more studies, ones that link vaccines, or some type of direct assault on the nervous system due to heavy metal toxicity, to Autism Spectrum Disorder specifically:

- Authier, F.J., et al. "Central nervous system disease in patients with macrophagic myofasciitis". *Brain*. May 1, 2001. Vol. 124, Iss. 5, pp. 974-983. Oxford University Press. Web. Feb. 11, 2015

This study examines neurological complications in patients who developed Macrophagic Myofasciitis (MM), a newly identified disorder in France and several western countries. It was found that MM is a direct result of aluminum-containing intramuscular vaccines. Of the 92 people that were identified with MM, 8 showed symptoms. This study details the symptoms of seven of those people which include chronic muscle pain, fatigue, central nervous system disorders, and cognitive or behavioral disorders.

> - Singh, V., K., et al. "Abnormal measles-mumps-rubella antibodies and CNS autoimmunity in children with autism". *Journal of Biomedical Science*. July/Aug 2002. Vol. 4, Iss. 9, pp. 359-364. Karger Publishers. Web. Feb. 12, 2015

This study found abnormally high measles antibodies in 75 of 125 children with ASD. More than 90% of the 125 children were also found to be positive for antibodies to myelin basic protein, or MBP. which is vital to the normal development of nerve tissue. This suggests that the autoimmune response is strongly associated with the MMR vaccine and that it contributed to the development of ASD.

> - Delong, Gayle. "A positive association found between autism prevalence and childhood vaccination uptake across the U.S. population". *Journal of Toxicology and Environmental Health, Part A*. 2011. Vol. 74, Iss. 14, pp. 903-916. Informa Healthcare. Web. Feb. 12, 2015

A positive association between ASD and vaccination was found by regression analysis and controlling for family income, ethnicity, and the relationship between the proportion of children who received the recommended vaccines by age two. The presence of speech or language impairment was also examined. Data from each state was obtained for these populations between 2001 and 2007.

- Nataf, Robert, et al. "Porphyrinuria in childhood autistic disorder: Implications for environmental toxicity". *Toxicology and Applied Pharmacology*. July 15, 2006. Vol. 214, Iss. 2, pp. 99-108. Elsevier B.V. Web. Feb. 12, 2015.

269 children with neurodevelopmental and related disorders were seen at a clinic in Paris between 2002 and 2004. 106 of them had ASD. All of the children who presented with ASD tested positive for coproporphyrin in the urine, and this finding was compared to a control group. Coproporphyrin is a natural byproduct of the breakdown of red blood cells. However, another form of this byproduct not natural to the body, precoproporphyrin, was also elevated. Precoproporphyrin is a tell-tale sign of heavy metal toxicity. Some of the autistic children were then treated with oral chelation using dimercaptosuccinic acid (DMSA), which significantly reduced the level of precoproporphyrin. This confirmed the suspicions that the autistic children were indeed exposed to high levels of environmental toxins from heavy metals.

- Kern, Janet, K., Jones, Anne, M. "Evidence of toxicity, oxidative stress, and neuronal insult in autism". *Journal of Toxicology and Environmental Health, Part B*. Nov./Dec. 2006. Vol. 9. Iss. 6, pp. 485-499. Taylor & Francis Group, LLC. Web. Feb. 12, 2015

This is an exhaustive study of obvious biomedical changes found in children that prove there was "neuronal cell damage or death sometime after birth as a result of insult." Examples of nerve damage included loss of Purkinje cells (cells found in the cerebellum which play a key role in motor coordination) and enlarged brains. In addition to neurological damage, abnormalities were also found in the immune and digestive systems. It was also observed that a decrease in glutathione coupled with an increase in oxidative stress apparently plays a key role in the physiology of certain underlying causes of autism. Glutathione is a naturally-occurring antioxidant responsible for the removal of toxic metals from body cells.

> - James, S.J., Slikker, W., III, et al. "Thimerosal Neurotoxicity is Associated with Glutathione Depletion: Protection with Glutathione Precursors". *Neurotoxicology*. Jan 2005. Vol. 26, Iss. 1, pp. 1-8. Elsevier B.V. Web. Feb. 12, 2015

This study states, "Although thimerosal has been recently removed from most children's vaccines, it is still present in flu vaccines given to pregnant women, the elderly, and to children in developing countries." The study also states, "Based on the known toxicity of methylmercury (a toxic byproduct of thimerosal metabolism), the cumulative ethylmercury exposure to U.S. pediatric populations in thimerosal-containing vaccinations was re-examined in 1999 and was found to exceed EPA recommended guidelines." Although nerve damage does result in lower levels of glutathione, it is suggested that the neurotoxin-caused depletion can be avoided by pretreatment with 100 micrograms of glutathione ethyl ester or N-acetylcysteine before vaccinating.

These are just 6 of 124 studies and reports that were collected by Ginger Taylor, an autism advocate and activist whose son developed autism after receiving his "required"

18-month vaccines. Many facts about vaccination adversities can be researched on the website of the National Vaccine Information Center, a nonprofit organization founded in 1982 dedicated to the prevention of vaccine injuries and deaths through public education. One of its co-founders, Barbara Loe Fisher, became an activist when her oldest son became afflicted with numerous learning disabilities after receiving a DPT vaccine. Thanks to those who have experienced the damage that vaccination can do firsthand, the word is spreading to inform others that there really is no such thing as a truly "safe" vaccine.

One must ask, then, how healthy is the unvaccinated population in comparison to the vaccinated? According to Dr. Tom Insel, former head of the Inter-Agency Autism Coordinating Committee, doing such a study to find out would be "unethical," as he reported on August 3, 2009 to the Senate Committee on Appropriations' hearing on autism. Therefore, we have to take a look at independent voluntary surveys, most of which occur outside the U.S., to find answers. One organization that has conducted such surveys is the International Medical Council on Vaccination, an association of medical doctors, registered nurses and other qualified medical professionals whose purpose is to counter the messages asserted by pharmaceutical companies and by governmental and medical agencies declaring vaccines as safe and effective. It is quite clear, after reading through their surveys and reports, that unvaccinated children are *far* healthier than the vaccinated population.

On April 1, 2016, the general public got its first good dose of vaccine-dangers truth when the movie *VaxXed: From Coverup To Catastrophe* was released. After all the backlash Dr. Andrew Wakefield received for his tireless exposing of the devastating impact of vaccine-induced injury on the lives of countless innocent children and the parents who have to care for them, he emerged from it all in a big way when he teamed up with Emmy-award winning producer Del Bigtree to make this movie. *VaxXed* speaks specifically about how the Centers for Disease Control and Prevention (CDC) deleted tons of data proving there is a link between the onset of autism, along with other severe neurological disorders, and the Measles-Mumps-Rubella vaccine. The families of several of the victims are interviewed, and the whistle-blower who exposed the cover-up, CDC scientist Dr. William Thompson, is seen as a hero.

Although the movie has been met with much resistance from mainstream media and health care-related organizations, the good work of educated parents, doctors, medical insiders, and the VaxXed National Tour bus has spread the truth widely and quickly. The film currently shows in private screening events around the country, and it can be purchased and streamed online. The film has led to the creation of many community activist groups, and invites are being received from around the globe for the truth about vaccine-induced injury to be told. Other works are currently on the drawing board by the same production team. Thanks to the driving campaign energized by seekers of the truth, more and more people are waking up. One can only hope and pray that there will be a day when we will never have to fear that another child may lose his or her life, or life in a state of health and happiness, because of a thoughtlessly-delivered vaccine.

8

Atlas Shifted

In January 2012, I presented my autism seminar at the Anoka-Hennepin School District in Anoka, Minnesota. After the program, a woman with Asperger's Syndrome approached me and asked if I could help her using the Upper Cervical Specific technique I talked about in my lecture. She told me she had a rather severe form of anxiety for which she was being medicated. She was also seeing a social worker regularly for ongoing counseling. The very next week, she came to see me in my office. Sure enough, I found that she had a rotated Atlas, which is the topmost vertebra of the spine. After her very first adjustment, she reported that she started sleeping normally for the first time in ages. Over the next several weeks, during which she visited me once per week, other symptoms improved including her anxiety. She noted such a dramatic improvement that she was able to almost totally discontinue her anti-anxiety medication. A few weeks later, I received a letter from her social worker commending me on my work.

In February 2014, I presented the same seminar at U3: Body, Mind, & Spirit, which was still located in Kutztown at the time. In attendance was the mother of a moderate-functioning adult who had many tics and who needed constant supervision. She became so intrigued by the information I presented that she started bringing her son to see me. Again, after just the first visit, during which I realigned a subluxated Atlas, he experienced remarkable improvement. His sleep had returned to normal so quickly that he was able to stop taking his prescription sleep medication altogether. He also went from having several outbursts a week to having very few. As I continued to see him over the next couple months, other improvements in his behavior were noted as well as with his level of concentration.

In both of these situations, nothing "magical" happened. I merely corrected the source of a nerve impingement, one that had existed perhaps since birth, one which nobody knew about since these people had never been to a chiropractor before. During my internship and earliest years in practice, I came to realize how prevalent upper cervical subluxations are, in congruence with Dr. Abraham Towbin's study on birth trauma. Therefore, I decided to make it an imperative part of what I do to pay particular attention to this part of the spine in all of my patients and clients. When you realize the magnitude of importance of all the nerves of the body that pass through the upper cervical spine, including the Vagus nerves and the bulk of the nerves that make up the spinal cord itself, it becomes apparent how vital to healthy living it is to keep this part of the spine aligned. This area is of such significance that Dr. Bartlett J. Palmer, the developer of chiropractic, referred to the Atlas as "the switch between man and God." With that philosophy, he perfected a technique specifically for the realignment of the Atlas and its adjoining bones, the Axis (C2 vertebra) below and the Occiput (back of the skull) above.

Over the years, I've helped people with a myriad of problems simply by adjusting the Atlas, moving it back into its proper position. The first time I ever did such a thing was when I saw my very first patient ever as a student intern working in the outpatient clinic in October 1997. With just *one* Atlas adjustment, a man in his 30s was instantly relieved of his excruciating nerve pain attacks from Trigeminal Neuralgia. Trigeminal Neuralgia is one of the most painful of chronic conditions known for which there is no cure. It often results in the patient committing suicide simply to escape the constant torture. That patient's painful episodes stayed away completely for two whole months. When they did return, the severity was nowhere near as debilitating as it was previously. In the years that followed, I helped people with ear infections, vertigo, colic, digestion problems, sleep problems, sinus problems, difficulty concentrating, temper control issues, headaches, irregular menses, and even blurred vision, just to name a few, simply by adjusting the upper cervical spine, most often the Atlas.

That's not to say that I adjust only the upper cervical spine, as many Upper Cervical Specific chiropractors do. I examine and realign the entire skeletal framework where and when needed. I often find, though, that many repeat and chronic problems, even with one's structural alignment itself, can be reversed when the upper neck region is paid close attention to. The main reason why a person's structural alignment may be affected is because the upper cervical spine contains an abundance of proprioceptor nerves, and these are easily impinged upon by an upper cervical subluxation. Proprioceptors regulate the body's balance and one's sense of position. When one of the upper cervical bones becomes subluxated, or misaligned, the impingement on the nerves may be so great that a loss of normal balance, vertigo, or abnormal gait or posture may result. In any case, misalignments of any bone in the skeletal framework can often be traced back to an upper cervical subluxation.

It is imperative for me to point out that the various Upper Cervical Specific techniques used by a chiropractor *do not* involve the stereotypical twisting and racking maneuvers people usually associate with chiropractic adjustments. Instead, they consist of either a tap, toggle, or vectorial guiding with the base of the palm, a finger, or a stylus. Because of the lightness of these maneuvers, I use the same approach when adjusting most of the rest of the spine. In reality, the brute force, twisting and turning, and jumping on top of someone to move their bones is almost never needed. For pediatric patients and for people who are already in great pain, these techniques are contraindicated entirely as they could cause more harm than good. It behooves me when I meet a fellow Doctor of Chiropractic who insists on showing off his "skill" by using such harshness. The late Dr. George Sabo, a chiropractor who took care of me between 1988 and 1992, once told me, "When you have your hands right on top of the bone that needs to move and you are pushing in the right direction, very little force is ever needed." I took that word of advice to heart, and my patients have always appreciated the outcome.

So, how is it that so many body systems could be affected when Atlas shifts? The biggest factor is the direction in which Atlas has moved. When Atlas is measured in a three-dimensional plane, there are more than a dozen different directions in which it could become misaligned. Depending on which, different nerves will be affected, all of which innervate, control, and regulate various parts of the body. Another factor is subjectivity. No two people are exactly alike. Two people with the same Atlas subluxation may not experience the same problem. Other factors to consider are how long Atlas had been out of alignment, the patient's tolerance level, and how much nerve impingement is being produced. Dr. Seth Sharpless, a neuropsychologist at the University of Colorado, proved that merely 10 mm Hg pressure, or the weight of a dime, placed on a nerve is enough to cause a nerve to lose 60% of its function if the pressure is maintained for 15 minutes[51]. That is significant! And when this pressure is prolonged enough to where people start experiencing symptoms such as pain, loss of normal function of a body system, or any of the problems previously mentioned, the most reliable and safe way for this process to be reversed is to have the pressure removed by way of a specific adjustment performed by a chiropractor.

While this may make it evident how physical symptoms can arise, it still leaves the question as to how people with autism can be helped. Much of what we discussed so far had to do with nerve impingement affecting organ systems along the distribution of involved nerves. But this isn't all that is affected. The nerves *above* the site of the misalignment are also impacted. According to Dr. David D. Palmer, the founder of chiropractic, pressure being placed on a nerve by a misaligned bone results in the tone of that nerve being changed. There is a tightening or loosening of the normal amount of nerve tension that causes either an excess or a reduction of nerve impulse (vibration) respectfully which in turn causes an over-functioning or under-functioning of the innervated organs[52]. Since impulses originate in the brain, a change in nerve tone directly affects the functioning of the brain itself. This is especially so if the site of nerve impingement is in the upper cervical spine.

Imagine there is too much vibration in the brain, as seen in anxiety or insomnia. On the other hand, imagine there is too little vibration, as there is with many learning disorders and sluggish processing. If there is an upper cervical subluxation present, then correcting the misalignment will restore normal nerve tone and improve brain function. Scientifically, we know now that this "vibration" Dr. Palmer was referring to is actually the exchange of charged ions along the course of a nerve. If the subluxation has been corrected and symptoms persist, or if there is not a subluxation to begin with, then one can assume that the most likely cause for symptoms is due either to a limitation of matter (injury or abnormal structure) or a pathological (disease-caused) distribution of neurotransmitters (chemical messengers found within the brain and nervous system). In these cases, medical intervention is necessary.

"Medical intervention" does not mean that prescription medications are always required. Herbal remedies given by a homeopath or a Doctor of Naturopathy could do just as well. For example, a study done in 1999 showed that an 800 mg. dose of Saint John's Wort is just as effective as a 20 mg. dose of Prozac[53]. Also, providing vibration from putative energy medicine practices, e.g. Reiki, Therapeutic Touch, etc., had been shown to promote healing for people with mild memory and behavioral disorders[54]. The healing possibilities offered by alternative medicine practices are only now beginning to be realized and studied. I am excited about the prospects for the future as more and more medical clinics and hospitals embrace Complementary and Alternative Medicine (CAM) therapies by creating entire departments dedicated to their practice and education. This integration and acceptance is making an impact in eroding away the age-old fables of such practices being anti-science or "the work of the devil."

9

Evolution of Consciousness

There are various theories and hypotheses that describe autism as an evolutionary process. Within the realm of science, arguments such as the extreme male brain theory and the imprinted brain theory suggest that fetal testosterone and genomic imprinting (respectively) are the reasons why certain traits develop in autism. I will focus less on science in this chapter and more on consciousness itself as a spiritually-evolving entity, or as the Reverend Noel McInnis puts it, "A re-education of our human sensibilities." After browsing many articles and perusing a few more, I've come to realize that there isn't a single author out there, as far as I know, who I can echo or even emulate in this discussion.

The evolution I am referring to is discussed in the teachings of the oldest known scriptures on Earth, the Vedas, particularly the Rg Veda, and similar texts such as the Upanishads and Puranas. These teachings also include the principle of living many lives, or reincarnation. To better understand the meaning of the evolution of consciousness and how it relates to autism, it is important to be aware of the concept of balance of forces, as in the fight between good and evil and the equalization of yin and yang energies. This concept is spoken of with the greatest of detail in the Tao Te Ching, one of the chief texts of Taoism. It is also spoken of in more recent writings of the late Dr. Wayne Dyer and in the book *A Unique Sufi Interpretation of Decoding the Quran* by Ahmed Hulusi. One must also know that the entire physical universe as we know it is based on the principle of duality.

According to Vedanta, one of the orthodox schools of Hindu philosophy, there is one God, and that God has manifested as the entire Universe. Why? Simply to experience Him/Herself for His/Her own amusement. This could have happened only by creating duality, that is the manifested physical world and the unmanifested consciousness that enlivens it. Therefore, we have opposites. Just as there cannot be day without night, male without female, positive without negative, there will *always* be evil in the world kept in check proportionally by the good. It is all synergistic. If God had never become manifest, there would only exist advaita, or the pure essence of God.

The balance of powers in duality is kept by the divine Source which has manifested as the multitudes. When evil begins to raise its ugly head, the living saints arise in this world to match the force. In this same way, as people are straying from their basic human principles of being, those who see things as they are will arrive just in time to keep society from becoming completely corrupted. They will present great intuition and creativity in this world. They come bearing the gifts of an elevated awareness, spiritual conflux, grounding of human reciprocity, and a deepening of interpersonal communication. This is why there are so many people with autism. However, only when people recognize their purpose for being here and learn how to interact with such an intellectual will their gifts bear fruit.

The autie's consciousness has evolved through countless lifetimes of learning. Now, being in this world but not of it, they need to figure out how to interact with it. Nonverbally at first, or perhaps precociously communicative and not well understood, they go about absorbing everything. They are still inside themselves, and they prefer to be there most the time. It is when they feel the absolute necessity to project themselves outward that they finally do so. They are peacemakers. They are nonviolent, contrary to what some people and the media make them out to be. They are perfectly human yet completely "other." Their brains process the universe in accentuated yet irrational ways. Because of this, they see it in ways the "normal" person could never imagine. Because the "normal" cannot imagine, they see the autie as some "thing" that needs correcting and disciplining. They fail to see the beauty in the gifts. Instead, they focus on why this creature is something totally different, not right, and an object of much-perceived burden.

How often are you surprised by the unexpected good deed or insightful words shared by a person with autism? What does *your* conscience tell you when you are face to face with such a being whom you cannot understand? What is your response when they tell you they feel as though they've been born on the wrong planet? The closed-hearted will attack them as though they are an invading alien species. When this happens, auties loses sight of their power and significance in this world. They are, after all, human and are therefore just as subject to physical and psychological pain as any neurotypical (person without autism). Those who take the time to connect in a loving and supporting way will help unlock the autie's full potential. As a result, their value to society will eventually become manifest. It is the parent, teacher, mentor, and advocate who believes this who will open the doors through which the autie will become all that he can be. When all is said and done, many will feel the shower of blessings upon them, all in the name of good — good that wards off evil, keeping it at bay to maintain a state of balance.

The autie is to be counted among the earthly angels, leaders, influencers, saints, and philosophers. It is because this world is in dire need of a new vision, a new perspective, a better way of functioning, that they are here in large numbers. It's not that they were born autistic; they came into this world with the potential of becoming so. They also came with the karma that allowed them the strength to bear the gifts they bring. They *are* the change that is needed, and they will make it all right. They are not dissonants to be medicated away or quashed by the unwinnable pursuit to make them blend into the very society they came here to change. Watch as they figure out for themselves how to blend, for everything they touch will be enlivened and renewed. This is a process to be celebrated, praised, and encouraged. In the end, they will give *you*, their strongest allies and supporters, all the credit. When allowed to blossom in their own time and in their own way, the world itself will reap the benefits of their actions. We are here to help you see this world and your own self in a way you never could have imagined without that brilliant vision we bring into this world.

And so, the process continues, more radiantly than ever.

10

What Happened in Arizona

For 285 days of my life, from June 25, 2012 until April 24, 2013, I lived in Yuma, Arizona. I wrote about all the events leading up to my move and why I chose Yuma in my first book. What I didn't mention were the details of the surrealness of the experience and the freedom I felt to act uncharacteristically for an autistic INFJ. Call it part of a midlife crisis if you wish, but it was really an attempt to reinvent myself. After growing up with so much self-doubt, after all the bullying I encountered both as a child and as an adult, after isolating myself on purpose for too long, after all the illnesses, after all the professional struggles, after being in an unfulfilling marriage for nearly ten years, after hearing all of my family's imposing expectations of me, I finally had enough. It really *was* time for a regeneration. And what a better place to do it than where I could see the Earth from horizon to horizon without obstruction, where I could feel my lungs expanding without limits. Yuma will go down as the best place I ever lived in regards to how free I felt. It is also the best place I ever lived in regards to my physical well-being.

I experienced just a small taste of what living in the desert would be like when I flew to Phoenix on May 30th to take the state board exam for my chiropractic license. When I stepped off the plane at the Sky Harbor International Airport that afternoon and experienced the 108-degree heat for the first time, my first thought was, "I'm almost home!" I felt as though I was being instantaneously healed. It was so comforting. It was just what I needed. I then looked forward all the more to living in Yuma. My overall health certainly needed to improve. Having sinus problems and sleep issues was my norm. When that desert air hit me, I knew change was imminent. As I walked through the airport, rode the taxi to my hotel, and settled into my hotel room, I felt an air of confidence come over me unlike any I had ever felt before. Arizona was definitely welcoming me with open arms.

The next morning, I woke up earlier than expected. I felt more refreshed than I thought I would. It was unusual to not have to go through several tissues during the night because of a runny nose. Once I was showered and ready for the day, I walked out into the desert heat simply to stand there and let it all hit me. I stood by the hotel's swimming pool just for a moment. Again, the heat poured through me as if it were healing me. During the rest of the day, both before and after the exam, I took every chance I could to spend time in the dry, healing sunshine. I really didn't want to go back to Pennsylvania. I never wanted to be in Pennsylvania in the first place. I ended up going there after filing for my divorce so that I could take care of my dad whose health was failing. Now I was just tasting Arizona for a day and then returning to be with my parents for what seemed like a continuing eternity.

It wasn't until twenty-three days later when I was finally on my way to Arizona for good. At first, the move seemed long and boring, being fueled only by the excitement over the possibilities of what lies at the end of the rainbow. Once I reached the New Mexico state line, I could feel my sinuses draining in an immense way. Years of chronic buildup was being eliminated in an instant. It was even hard to take a breath at times because of how much junk was in my throat. I took this to be a great sign, and I prayed for the healing to continue. That it surely did! By the time I got to the other end of the state, I was breathing the best I ever had in my life. The desert was already proving how powerful its effects would be in my life. I was amazed and in awe. I felt that I had made the best possible move by wanting to be in this part of the country. But the best was yet to come.

It was about 7:00 in the evening on Monday, June 25 when I first set foot on Yuman soil. After pulling off Interstate 8, my first stop was the parking lot of Dillard's at the Yuma Palms Regional Center. I turned the air conditioner off, opened the windows, and was immediately greeted by the same 108-degree heat that I basked in during my one-day visit to Phoenix three weeks earlier. But this was different. There was a degree of sophistication to it. The pen was now to the paper, and the real journey had begun. As I drove around, I immediately felt intimidated by the size of the city. It was so spread out, very unlike what I was used to seeing growing up in the northeast. For a city with a population just over 90,000, I was expecting to see a large centralized area. Instead, there were many types of neighborhoods scattered throughout a 100-square-mile area. Destiny could take me anywhere, and no one place looked ideal. In fact, I actually felt more lost than I thought I would.

I figured that before I started to look for a place to live, I should get to know the different areas first. I had an inkling, thanks to articles and forums I had read through, that the Fortuna Foothills area located just to the east of the city line was the nicer place to be, away from the congestion and what city life there was. I planned to go there the next day since it was already late in the evening. I drove around the downtown areas before getting a room at the Super 8 Motel on 16th Street. I also called a guy named David whom I had contacted online in order to get to know more about the area. He lived in the Foothills, and we made plans to meet the next day. While I was in my hotel room, I looked through listings in the local newspapers and on the internet to get an idea of what apartments were out there. There were very few, which surprised me given the population of the city. The ones that were available were not in any areas I was interested in. I was starting to look more and more forward to the next day's drive through the Foothills and to meeting David.

At the same time that I was excited about starting my new life, my heart was aching over the fact that shortly after leaving for my cross-country trip my dad had been admitted yet again to the hospital. Being in and out of hospitals had been a regular thing for him during my two-and-a-half-month stay in Pennsylvania. This, we figured, would be just another one. From that point on, I checked in with my family on a daily basis to receive updates about my dad's condition. This visit started out as just another bout, but his condition became graver by the day. I've seen people bounce back from some pretty amazing things over the years. I was certain that my dad would do the same because of how strong he always was. He had the will and the drive to keep going. People who do not have such a will are the ones who decline rapidly, even from less-serious illnesses. Having seen this for myself as a health care provider was a great lesson in how the power of the mind and the determination to survive can bring a person through just about anything. I was continuing to be optimistic, as was my mom, during this most recent admission.

I had booked my stay at the Super 8 Motel for the next three nights since I wasn't sure how long it would be before I found a place to live. I also figured it would be nice to be able to sleep in after such a long drive without being concerned about needing to check out by a certain time. That first night in Yuma, I fell asleep well before midnight which is an unusual feat for me since I am a devout night owl. I slept soundly through the night. When I woke up the next morning, I was amazed at how great I felt. It was also good to see that I was able to wake up at a decent time in the morning. Being a night owl goes hand in hand with being a late sleeper. That certainly wasn't the case on *this* day. I got myself ready, and I headed straight to the Foothills. I drove fourteen miles, all the way to South Foothills Boulevard, where my station wagon broke down. Unknowingly, it had been handed a death sentence just before I left Pennsylvania when I had the transmission flushed and filled. Nobody ever told me to never do this to a vehicle with high mileage. Now I needed a new transmission, and I had to continue making my way around in a rental car.

My planned get-together with David was anything but promising. I contacted him as I was driving to the Foothills. When my car broke down, I called him again to let him know where I was and to see if he could help me. Although he did, I was quite dismayed to find him to be quite the opposite of the spiritually advanced person he led on to be. He was belligerent and insulting, to say the least. It was a blow to my expectation that I would be meeting all sorts of enlightened people in the desert. It ultimately occurred to me, as time went on, that the spiritualists I met there were all just as lost and hypocritical as many I had met over the years. Although I never contacted David again after that day, he did give me one good memory — my first good view of an amazing desert sunset, the first of countless to come during the next ten months. That took place in the vastness among the hills just behind where he lived in the Foothills Mountain Estates neighborhood. He also gave me my first real opportunity to stand up for myself and demand something better (other than getting divorced, that is) when I called him that night to let him know that I did not deserve to be treated like an imbecile and that our "friendship" was no longer in the cards.

Only two days after arriving in Yuma, I was told my dad had worsened to the point where he wasn't expected to live much longer. My hopefulness along with the positive picture my mom had been painting kept me believing I would not have to make such an early return. But the story from Damon was very different, which made me wish I had not yet left for Arizona. I did promise before I left to return in the fall when dad was to have a heart operation just like the one I had. That evening, though, I made my travel plans to fly back to Pennsylvania. Before I even got on the airport shuttle at 8:00 the next morning, I received the phone call from Damon telling me that dad passed away. Building a new life in the desert was suddenly put on hold. The return home for dad's funeral was not a pretty one. Among all the obvious sadness were the words of condemnation from my brothers over my whole Arizona expedition and "abandoning" dad. When I returned to Yuma ten days later, I felt relieved to be back in the healing heat. I was naturally sad, though, knowing that the family member who supported me and believed in me the most was no longer there.

As I drove around the city and met more people, the feeling of being overwhelmed and intimidated wore away, slowly but surely. Yes, meeting and conversing with people came easier simply because I put myself out there with a free and upbeat spirit without judgment of myself or anyone else. I was a clean slate in an unspoiled land. I drove to the various parts of the city, both the good and the bad, and I talked to people every place I stopped. After all, Yuma was my new home, and I was sure to make my relocation worth the while. I was there to find a new potential, a new height, and to finally experience professional success as predicted by my astrocartograph.

One might wonder how I was able to hold myself together through all of this. The travel, being in a strange place, knowing nobody, the car breaking down, my dad passing away, the betrayal of a new friend. Many people with autism might find these things devastating enough to drive them into a deep withdrawal or depression. But change was just a natural part of life I got used to over the years. Road trips were nothing new to me with all the traveling to the New Jersey shore I did with my family as a youngster, trips throughout New England while visiting my uncle Valent in New Hampshire, and big moves to Indiana, Georgia, Kentucky, Minnesota, and now Arizona. Losing friends was par for the course over the years, so that too was nothing new. Also, I had already developed the ability to hold myself together well, thanks to all my health challenges throughout my life. And when news came that my dad had passed away, my knowing that death is merely a change of venue, whereby we pass from this world back to the spirit dimension, helped me to feel at ease. I guess you could say experience was my best teacher. As Bob Marley once said, "You never know how strong you are until being strong is your only choice." Now I felt that the whole reason why I was even there in Arizona was to take the next step in my spiritual evolution.

I soon found a room to rent in a very nice home in the Castle View neighborhood. But looks were deceiving. After living for three weeks with the crazy cat lady who was stealing my mail, I finally found a very nice and affordable mobile home in the Foothills Country Club Estates area, thanks to the help of another person I got to know online before moving to Yuma. For two-and-a-half months, that cozy little trailer on East 38th Street was more than just my home. It was an ideal meditation cave. Because most of the Foothills is asleep and closed up during the summer, only to become alive and quite busy during snowbird season, my entire being was cast into a much-welcome state of rest and quietude. I spent many a night on the trailer rooftop, lying on my back and staring up at the stars. At the same time, the vastness of the view and the eeriness of the desert around me gave me the sensation that my entire consciousness was expanding. It was as if I was being prepared for some kind of transformation. In due time, it became quite chilling and otherworldly to realize just how true this was.

I finally received my chiropractic license on July 16th, and on August 16th I saw my first patient. During the next eight months, I ended up with thirty-seven patients. Only five of them saw me on a regular biweekly basis. This was indeed the fastest a practice had ever grown in all the places I ever lived. However, it was not enough to pay any rent anywhere. I did, however, have a nice bit of pocket change during the busier times to buy food and gas with. It was also just enough for buying a coffee at the Starbucks at 16th Street & Pacific Avenue where I spent my days with my laptop, using the internet and typing. One day in August, I decided to buy a newspaper to check out the local happenings. I figured becoming active in the community would be the best way for me to make contact with people. Although this plan seemed contrary to what an introverted autie would do, it was something I *had* to do. I was not only there to enjoy a sense of freedom but also to try to build a business no matter how bad I was at it. I was there to reinvent myself, not to hide away from the world or to do and be the same ol' same ol'. I came across an ad for Wednesday evening spaghetti dinners at the local AmVets post in the Foothills. When I went there for the first time the following Wednesday, I had no idea how instrumental the people I met there would become to the rest of my days of living in Yuma.

The AmVets soon became my place of refuge, my home away from home. Throughout my life, I always found it easy to associate with people who were much older than me, accepting adults who always seemed eager to listen to a wise and respectable youngster. The people at the AmVets were no exception. While contact with people in my own age bracket was limited to my patients and the baristas at Starbucks, the people at the AmVets made me feel more at home than I ever did anywhere else I lived. I could always find someone to chat with there. Eventually, I was eating dinner there almost every night of the week. It was easy for me to come out of my shell whenever certain people were around, mainly Bonnie Rothi and her husband Charlie. I also now had a place where I could volunteer my time to a worthy cause either by working in their kitchen or selling poppies at the local supermarkets.

Some nights were much busier than others at the AmVets, especially during snowbird season. When I felt the need to escape from the crowd for a moment, since crowds weren't really my thing anyway, I simply walked outside into the patch of desert behind the building. That spot was just as good as any for me to watch the sunset or to look up at the stars. As my time in Yuma wore on, I found myself spending more and more time in that patch of desert, contemplating my growing hardships and disappointment over not being able to find stability. During my hard times, it was because of people I met at the AmVets who bought me dinner and who let me live at their place when I had nowhere else to go. The brunt of my hardships all started at the end of September when I could no longer afford to live in the motor home on East 38th Street.

While still enjoying life in the mobile home, I figured I'd try my hand at dating. Having been off the market for more than ten years, and not being very good at it anyway, I was very unsure of myself. I met a girl named Cheryl through a free online dating website. We went out on three dates, but there was no communication in between. Despite sending her texts and calling her on occasion, she never reciprocated unless she wanted to go out. She seemed very ordinary, and she had no ambitions in life. After those three dates, I stopped communicating with her altogether. I needed depth. I was beyond ordinary, and I needed a partner who walked a similar spiritual road. That got me thinking about all those years ago when I was single. I was single for the very same reason — because I needed to experience some sort of common ground *first* before ever pursuing a relationship. Unlike the usual way things progress for the average person, it is more an INFJ thing rather than an autism trait whereby a deep connection needs to be found. Casual chit chat that seems to lack substance leads to rapid ends of any kind of romantic interest[55]. I found that, even now, my nature and my desires had not changed.

Eventually, I did strike up the interest with Barbara that was much fodder for my first book. Although trying to turn that casual online friendship into a romantic relationship was destined to fail, the sending and receiving of ethereal communication between us opened a whole new realm to the already-eerie air in the desert. By the time that relationship began, the initial depth and intrigue I felt when I first arrived in Yuma had all but disappeared amidst my struggles. The level of connection I had with Barbara rekindled the fascination so much that I felt I was getting my spiritual revival back on track.

When the cooler weather came around sometime after the end of summer, I made it a regular exercise to venture out on foot into the desert to meditate. During the same period of time, I learned from people at the AmVets about great places locally I could drive to in order to admire the desert sunset. Though it was apparent that Arizona was treating me well despite my difficulty becoming settled, a rift was developing as the relationship with Barbara continued. What finally ended the whole Barbara saga was when I expressed the fact that having a stable relationship with her was more important to me than being on a quest in the desert. I was willing to give it all up and to return to Pennsylvania to be with her. After all, it just seems nonsensical to have a long-distance relationship in which we'll never be together nor have any plans of permanency. She suddenly felt that she was intruding on my goals and disrupting my life journey. She was also startled by my eagerness to commit, so much so that she brought our relationship to an end.

The greatest memories of Yuma didn't even happen until the final two months I was there. In February 2013, a Denny's Restaurant and a Starbucks opened for business in the Foothills. They were game changers. No longer did I have to drive thirteen miles to the Starbucks at 16th & Pacific to do my writing. A regular late-night crowd rapidly formed at the new Denny's where I became good friends with the night manager, James Mann. These were also the months when I did most of my desert hiking. As I talked more to Bonnie and Charlie, I started becoming interested in joining them during their jeeping expeditions far out past the Gila Mountains. Ironically to the life I was creating for myself in the Foothills, I spent the month of March living in a room at a house in the Del Oro Mobile Estates off of South Avenue B in the downtown area, thanks to a friend from the AmVets gifting me with a month of rent. Because of all the positives that were starting to happen, though, I did not mind having to continue that long trek back and forth between downtown and the Foothills.

Whether lying on top of a trailer, hiking in the desert, or sitting somewhere to admire the sunset, one staple that was added to my routine was meditating. This gave rise to a new dimension of reality. The sun during the day and the moon at night were so vivid. They were like balls hanging on a Christmas tree that could be easily plucked from the sky. Throughout history, travelers through this part of Arizona had written great words about the sunsets and the night sky. During the late nights when I'd lie on the roof of my mobile home in the Foothills, I was taken in by mysterious lights that would streak across the sky. It became a regular practice for me to walk through the area of desert just south of the intersection of East 48th Street and Hunter Avenue, contemplating life's greatest mysteries as the sun set over the horizon. While meditating in my car at night, looking out into the desert while parked at the dark and quiet intersection of East 40th Street and South Avenida Compadres, I would often see peculiar lights suddenly appearing and standing motionless above me. Some people said they were military flares. But I knew they were not because I saw those too, and the difference was unmistakable.

On one particular night, March 1 at about 9:00 PM, I saw a bizarre flashing green light zipping back and forth across the desert. It appeared in three "waves," each wave lasting about ten seconds. The whole experience was definitely otherworldly, and it left me with a feeling of exhilaration and excitement over having witnessed an inexplicable desert phenomenon. I've heard that such things happen from time to time, and I felt privileged to have seen something so peculiar. Perhaps not coincidentally, it was during the next several days I felt overwhelming surges of chi energy opening my heart chakra and expanding my conscious awareness, literally. In an instant, I could be overcome with the feeling of an utter bliss that is usually only experienced in deep states of meditation. Or, I could be watching the actions of people I know and love who were far away, knowing what they were thinking and feeling at that precise moment. Abilities and blissfulness as such are commonplace for one who is spiritually advanced, as living gurus and Siddhas are. I will talk more about these qualities later in this book.

Even though things seemed to be getting exciting during February and March, my money woes actually became worse than ever. When business dried up as the snowbirds started to go back home, even eating and putting gas in my car became real struggles. During this time, I was also preparing to make a planned trip back to Pennsylvania to visit my mom for her birthday in April. Because I had been given only one month of rent for the house I lived in downtown, the big question was where I would be living upon my return. Thanks to Bonnie, she was keeping her eyes out for places for rent in the Foothills, which is where I preferred to live anyway. Thanks to James, the manager at Denny's, I had a job lined up as a dish washer to keep me afloat once I came back.

I was in Pennsylvania for sixteen days, from April 4th until the 20th. I figured this extended stay would be enough time for me to spend with my mom and say hi to some old friends. But because my heart and my head were in Arizona, I was only counting down the days until I would be there again. When I did arrive back in Yuma on the 20th, though, everything changed. A mobile home which Bonnie had found was rented out from under me. I also discovered that James no longer worked at Denny's, so I no longer had a job to come back to. Living in a homeless shelter became my only viable option. However, there were drawbacks to that plan, mainly the grossly uncomfortable sleep and bathroom schedules. Sleeping in one big room with countless other people on floor mattresses, and having to be up at a specific early-morning time for breakfast every day, would only make me outrageously miserable. That left me with only one solution, and that was to pack up everything and head back to Pennsylvania. I was praying for a miracle, but it never came.

I stayed in Yuma only four more days. I spent two nights sleeping in hotels, which wiped out all the rest of my money, and the next two nights sleeping in my station wagon behind the AmVets. I took my last two showers at two different truck stops. Now, all the money I had to my name was a $10 bill in my wallet and the $20 to keep my credit union account open. In the afternoon of April 24, I packed up all my belongings, which I had kept in a storage unit. I ate one last Wednesday evening spaghetti dinner at the AmVets, and then I let everyone there know that my days in Yuma were over. My drive back home began right then and there. The trip was being paid for by a credit card my parents had given me to use only in the case of an emergency. As I began the 2,600-mile trip back to Pennsylvania, I enjoyed one final view of the Gila Mountains and the Sonoran Desert. The return to the East Coast seemed twice as long as the trip I took to move to Arizona just ten months earlier. It didn't help to be driving the entire second half of the trip through an unrelenting downpour. It was as if all of Heaven itself was weeping for what became of my attempt to turn myself around.

It eventually occurred to me that Yuma did indeed give me everything the planet Jupiter promised. I had built a practice bigger and faster than I ever did before. In addition to the positive influence of Jupiter, the negative manifested as well, namely the fact that I was constantly unsettled. During my time there, I lived in seven different places, four of which I paid for with my own money, three of which I stayed in only as long as I could afford them. In two places, I lived a total of three-and-a-half months rent free. All I really would have needed was a place I could take a shower every day, and I might have stayed in Yuma. Living in my car didn't seem so bad for the two days that I did, but I really needed a roof over my head. Therefore, the only option was to go back to where my family was.

Yuma did give me exactly what I needed. I did well with pretending to be somewhat extroverted. I did talk to a wider variety of people when the conversations were upbeat and without depth. The spiritual encounters I had, between connecting with nature around me and witnessing the lights in the desert while meditating, were experiences I could not have grown without. There certainly must have been beings from other worlds around me, perhaps present to let me know that I was indeed on the right track. There indeed was a method to the madness, a vital process to my evolution. I got what I went there for. Now it was time for the majnun to go back to his homeland where he could finally make a difference. His years of wandering took him to the desert where he was given the realization of everything he ever needed: himself.

11

Beyond Awareness: Reaching the Next Spiritual Height

Jesus once said, "No man comes to my Father except by me." (Lamsa English Peshitta Bible, John 14:6) In the same way, Lord Krishna said, " I am the way, come to Me." Likewise, Guru Arjan Dev Ji, the fifth Guru of Sikhism, said, "They who fall at the Guru's feet are freed from bondage.....No one can save except the Guru." Other examples of the same declaration can be found in various religious and philosophical texts. But what does it really mean? It all means the same thing: that in order for one to gain the *experience* of God, as opposed to a knowledge-inspired awareness of God, the right path *must* be revealed by one who has consummated it. Because people with autism already vibrate on a higher spiritual level, ergo they are already hypersensitive to energy changes, they are typically closer to achieving that which many on the spiritual path may take years to accomplish. Once the *experience* of pure divine essence is encountered, one *automatically* sees the world differently. The desire to be "normal," or even to pretend to be neurotypical, is forever abandoned.

A truly enlightened master who knows the path to spiritual realization is definitely hard to find, even if you go looking for one. Such a guru does not seek to recruit devotees. Devotees somehow find the guru when the time is right. Also, a guru will not automatically tell you he's a guru. It's something you have to figure out for yourself. As for me, I was lucky enough to have met Dr. Ellen Bagetakos-Handlin in 1996. Ellen was a classmate of mine in chiropractic school who knew my life was in a rut that year. I was suffering momentary depression over a failed relationship, the Chronic Fatigue Syndrome was at its worst point, and other health concerns came to a head during this time which caused me to miss the entire summer term. Ellen told me about the guru she knew and about the spiritual path she walked. Despite Ellen's urging for me to meet her guru, I resisted for a whole two years. It wasn't until I met Betty McKeon in July of 1998 that I finally decided to meet this guru. As it turned out, Betty knew the same guru.

This guru's practice is a true, time-tested path that began in 1921 when a young boy named Krishna Rau met a living saint named Nityananda near the city of Mangaluru, India. This path was well depicted in Elizabeth Gilbert's biopic and book "Eat, Pray, Love." From the time I first visited the meditation center dedicated to this path in August of 1998, it took less than two months for me to be gifted with the power of spiritual awakening, or *Shaktipat*. Receiving this new vision does not make life easier. Your life may, in fact, become more difficult. Many people have the misconception that being "spiritual" means that your life is suddenly easy. That is not at all true. Shaktipat gives you a perception you never had before. You see things differently, and you learn from your experiences. To sum it up, as long as you stick with the routine, you will never be the same person. You *will* be better. The guru commences the inner transformation, and the rest is due to the movement of energy.

Inside everyone, two kinds of energy exist: the active chi and the typically dormant Kundalini. Chi is always in motion. It is what binds and keeps the entire Universe alive. It is the force behind the flowing of blood, the beating of the heart, the rushing of a river, the power of the wind, and the heat of the sun. It is ever-present, and it can never fade. It is our life force. The dormant Kundalini, in contrast, is said to be lying in wait at the base of the spine, ready to go to work upon its awakening through Shaktipat. Through acts of spiritual development and exercise such as yoga, praying, chanting, contemplation, etc., Kundalini is directed in the way she needs in order to bring a person to a state of spiritual perfection, or enlightenment. Through her movement, in an upward direction through the spine, the individual becomes pure in thought and intention. One often becomes healthier and adopts a lifestyle of wellness without much effort. Shaktipat, if given by someone who is *not* an enlightened being, can be quite dangerous. Only a saint, in the truest sense of the word, can safely give this gift and direct a student in the ongoing process of spiritual development.

When I received Shaktipat on October 3, 1998, I had no idea what had happened at that moment. It wasn't until I talked to Betty immediately after the program that I realized the magnitude of the event. I was sitting on the floor among the rest of the people in the meditation hall. We were chanting in the Sanskrit language, which is part of the regular gatherings, or satsangs. My entire consciousness suddenly went elsewhere. I lost all awareness of being in the room or of being anywhere at all. What I saw next was bedazzling. I witnessed the beginning of the universe, *the* Big Bang, as it actually happened. I watched as heavenly bodies flew past me. Over the next few seconds, my awareness gradually came back to the room. What followed during the next six months were bizarre, yet not scary, visions, dreams, and sensations during both my waking and sleeping states.

By sharing my experiences with my closest fellow yogis, I received validation that I had indeed been blessed by the guru. The only question was why so soon? People can chant, meditate, contemplate, and do seva (selfless services in the name of spiritual rightfulness) for years and not experience what I was fortunate enough to see. It wasn't until well after I was diagnosed with ASD in 2008 when I figured that it was all due to one thing, the fact that I was *already* vibrating on a higher level before ever visiting the yoga center. Vibrating on a higher level is also what I attributed my natural intuition to. All it took was one virtual touch by the guru to kick it up a notch and to take me to the next tier. I am also sure that vibrating on a higher level is why I am a natural at energy healing, as I discovered during my Reiki I and II training.

Although people with autism and the people who know them may feel as though they are far removed from being able to obtain anything so spiritually advanced, quite the opposite is true. As I pointed out earlier, people on the autism spectrum function on a higher vibrational frequency. But what does that mean, and how does this occur? "Vibration" is not how active or reactive the nervous system is. Nor is it how hyper a person may be. It is an etheric concept. When stringed instruments are played, the sounds they produce are caused by vibration when the string is struck. The greater the amount of vibration, the higher the sound. In the same way, everything in the Universe vibrates. Have you ever heard the saying that the entire universe has a certain sound to it? Vibration is directly related to movement. Raise the vibration of water, and it becomes steam. Lower the vibration, it turns to ice.

In a similar way, people have a certain vibration. Different people vibrate at different levels. Lower your vibration through negative thinking and lifestyle choices, and you invite illness and conflict. Raise your vibration through meditation, relaxation, and productivity, and you automatically become more spiritually-inclined and visionary. Awaken the dormant Kundalini and fuel it through disciplined spiritual activity, known in Sanskrit as *dharma*, and your vibration level supersedes that which a human is capable of achieving through ordinary means. Spiritual awareness, greater insight, intuition, inner peace, calmness, greater focus, and a greater capacity for innate healing all become natural states of being when vibrating at a higher level. Everyone is capable of such growth *without exception.*

The Shaktipat experience and the awakened Kundalini are not to be taken lightly. Let's take a lesson from Star Wars Episode V when the Jedi master Yoda was teaching young Luke Skywalker to become a fearless and powerful Jedi Knight. Yoda told Luke that he had to enter the Dark Side Cave in order to confront his greatest fear. When he did, it almost broke him down completely because he was suddenly made aware of the darkness within himself that needed to be conquered. His tenacity eventually brought him to be the victor over his own inner hauntings. In the same way, Kundalini brings each one of us into our cave where we must do battle with our own dark side, with that which can seem to overpower us. Our fears, aversions, vices, suppressed memories, subconscious tendencies, past traumas, and disappointments all come to the surface. We come face to face with them, and battle lines are drawn. If we see the process through, there is no way we can fail. Those who give up because of their skeletons will never reach the level of enlightenment they seek. This process is called, in the Hindu tradition, "purification of samskaras," or the burning away of everything that gives us our current beliefs, judgments, habits, likes and dislikes, and self-imposed limitations.

People in general tend to hide their past mistakes and traumatic events, such as abuse, and often resort to feelings of guilt and hurt. As Kundalini moves, these things are eventually erased. Thus, a person becomes liberated from all those chains. It is a *process*, one which takes most people many years to go through, especially if they vibrated at a very low level for most their life. For a person with autism, samskaras may be just as deep, just as ingrained in the mind. Because they naturally vibrate at a high level, the purification process, even though just as tedious and challenging, may not last as long. Feeling freer and experiencing greater clarity of mind are not too far off. Through understanding the process and stick-to-itiveness, they certainly can feel as though they climbed every mountain that stood in their way. Once you start to experience the nature of pure consciousness on the other side, there is no turning back. You can never return to those binds that held you back ever again.

The purification of samskaras may seem very odd to the non-yogi. There are actual physical effects that could, but not always, accommodate the process. No adverse problem can result from these effects when the Kundalini energy is directed by a true enlightened master. As Kundalini moves, different sensations may be felt in various areas of the body. One may feel heat, cold, or a buzzing sensation. These sensations are not unlike those felt during various poses in hatha yoga. Sometimes these feelings may be accompanied by the urge to shiver, shake, or even to have some sort of vocal outburst, events which are known as *kriyas*. Because one may be reliving unpleasant moments at the same time that they are feeling the sensations, people may become afraid and stop practicing their exercise altogether. It would be the equivalent of Luke Skywalker having emerged from the cave because of how unpleasant it was to be in there having never conquered his greatest fear. As time goes by, and as long as one continues his practices, the kriyas will diminish as the samskaras lose their grip.

As for me, I always look forward to the next time I do my favorite spiritual exercise, sitting to chant and then meditating afterward. During these activities, I go through the process of battling through samskaras and then floating on waves of bliss. It's not some New-Age concept that is being embraced. It is the promise written in a 2,400-year-old text known as the Bhagavad Gita whereby such a state is gifted to the disciple who places his entire focus, through all his thoughts and all his actions, on God. For a person with autism, finding freedom from identifying himself by the rules he makes for himself and by what he does in life is indeed emancipating. He is reformed. He is a new person. No, he doesn't suddenly become neurotypical. He becomes a person whose autism is his own best friend as well as the ally of everyone around him who notices the radiance of an untethered mind set in a divine light.

12

Turning an Old Leaf

In order for you to enjoy success in the future, you need to close the door to what didn't work for you in the past. Sometimes fate does that for you, as it had for me ever since my return to Pennsylvania. It's as if the Universe was telling me I couldn't go back to the life I once had. That included the people I once considered "friends." It all had to go. Something new was on the horizon, something better. I didn't know that at first. It all began in late July 2013, and it started with the person I considered to be my best friend. I've known Lisa since we were in kindergarten together. Because we had been classmates up until tenth grade, and since we remained in contact with each other off and on throughout our adult years, I felt as though I could tell her *anything*. I found out how very wrong I was.

On one particular day, I spoke intimately about my sexual likes and dislikes. Apparently, speaking to her about sex in an adultly appropriate way was too much for her. There wasn't a malicious thought in my head when I brought the topic up, as I knew she was happily married. Instead of telling me that she was uncomfortable with the topic, she completely shut me off and refused to talk to me any longer. The final nail in the coffin was when I asked her if she would respond in the same way to her autistic son if he one day talked about sex without filter or boundary considerations. A forty-five-year friendship was suddenly over. In the aftermath, I lost two friends we had in common. One of them was Michael, the person who got me interested in being a firefighter all those years ago.

Although it seemed a tragedy that I had lost the only friend I could talk to, less than three months later I met Becky. My social life continued to be on par since I continued to get together on an almost-weekly basis with a friend named Andre, whom I've known since I was in ninth grade. Andre and I would hang out together at either of two different restaurants. A couple times I even went to his house. He was impressed by Becky and Brittany, and he was happy for me. But in April of 2014, it was as if he simply vanished. He suddenly had no time for the regular routines and the friends he knew. I occasionally received messages from him saying that he became busy with duties he had taken on at his local fire department. Since we were still connected on social media, I saw when he would post pictures of himself with people at social events. I can't say this change was entirely out of character since it became apparent over time that we certainly walked different paths with opposite lifestyles.

My younger and naïve self would have thought that I had done something wrong, that I once again was a failure who nobody liked. Such a reaction is typical, in fact a hallmark, of someone who has autism. Yes, it is true that we lose contact with people and change friends over the course of our lifetime. Nobody is to blame for that. But it seemed that for me, the influence of the Universe was causing such a change to happen at an accelerated rate. Because of my spiritual maturation during the course of the past sixteen years at that point, I learned to see such losses as merely a change, a *gigo* effect, or "garbage in-garbage out" process.

I developed the ability to look at things objectively. Seeing the bigger picture helped me to realize that in order for me to achieve a greater awareness, that which limited my views had to be eliminated *first*. I was entering a new phase. This became quite evident as time went by in my relationship with Becky, with the people I met because of her, and in opportunities that came my way because of knowing her. They were exactly what I needed in order to reach my full potential. I never could have moved further up the mountain if I continued to be with people who had no plans on progressing.

Life is a continuous journey. Getting stuck in the "bubble" never leads anywhere. I first left Pennsylvania in 1992, which was a move that shocked everyone because of how attached I was to the bubble I was living in. Even my lifelong friend, Father Stephen Halabura, made note of the tremendous faith I had for leaving in hopes of finding something better. Because leaving the bubble was indeed the best thing I ever did, I was actually angry over having to return in order to have a roof over my head in April 2013. Despite the unfortunate return, the spiritual evolution didn't end. I had to remain outside the old bubble, and that process took care of itself. Because of all the people I met since my return, I developed a completely new life in the same geographical place I originated. Everything came full circle, and nothing went back to the way it was. It was as if I was prevented from regressing. My awareness of the big picture, of my seemingly-small part in the Divine's greater plan, kept me moving forward without skipping a beat.

It's a general idea in the conscience of most people that in order to change your life you have to change your location. In reality, and as the saying goes, wherever you go, there you are. Your life can make a complete 180-degree change in direction, and you can reinvent yourself, right where you already are. The key is you must *want* the change. I mentioned earlier that your life choices determine the level you vibrate at. Lower vibration will attract more low vibration. Higher vibration attracts more high vibration. Low vibration describes the life of content with the ordinary, gossip, indulging in vices, having no ambitions, feeling like a victim, feeling as though there is no room for improvement, and readily seeing and finding the faults in the world. High vibration is the opposite. You *know* that you are worthy of more, and your actions signify your readiness to find your greater potential. You take control of your own journey. You see the world as your teacher. You pray, you meditate, and you have faith while you perform rightful actions. You are open to receiving the grace of God. Should you be so blessed to come in contact with an enlightened being, it comes in the form of the awakened Kundalini which gives you a greater vision.

On November 12, 2014, I received the icing on the cake of all closures to the past. I was standing in line at a minimart in Sinking Spring, waiting to pay for my sandwich. A customer walked through the door, and I turned to look. My jaw hit the floor in an instant. It was the infamous Barbara, the one who was involved with from a distance during my days as a madman in the desert. I immediately realized what a poor decision it would have been for me to approach her at that moment. She had the most horrible, distant scowl on her face. I wasn't sure if it was because I was there or because that was her usual state of being. In any case, the words that went through my head were, "I can't believe I was once in love with such a miserable grump." Then I concluded how very lucky I was to not have any contact with her at all. She walked a distance from me and then disappeared into the restroom. I never saw her again.

Change doesn't happen overnight. In his book "Awakening the Giant Within," Anthony Robbins mentions that there is a lag time, a space between the moment you change your direction in life and the time when you finally start to see results. It requires only faith to stay the course during this lag time. Like with every new journey, the first step is always the hardest to make. Sometimes you need to take a blind leap of faith into the unknown. The path doesn't always reveal itself until after the first step has been taken. You don't even have to know where you're going. Unwavering faith in The Divine *always* takes you in the right direction. You can feel when inspiration fills you. You will feel it in your gut, literally. God is the one "speaking" when you feel that buzzing in your solar plexus area. *That's* the signal for you to follow a certain path, to perform a certain task, and to breathe life into a new possibility. It's really no great mystery. When your level of vibration is on par with that of the great Consciousness that makes up the entire Universe, you will have a level of knowingness that is undeniable. Although it cannot be understood and is often balked at by the ordinary person who lacks vision, *everyone* has this capacity. *Everyone* is connected to God in this way. God is the vine, and we are indeed the branches — undivided, inseparate, and nondual.

13

Changes

People with autism do not typically handle change very well. That's a given. But then again, many people, autistic or not, find it unpleasant. Why someone on the spectrum finds it extremely threatening is because they've become accustomed to a routine. It is more than just their comfort level which is at stake. They once again become burdened with the tremendous effort they had to go through to form ways to integrate themselves and learn to navigate the world in the first place. When that process is disrupted, and change is suddenly thrust upon them, it's as if you've thrown them into a river when they don't know how to swim. Panic is what surely causes them to have a meltdown or an outburst. Anger is certain to follow, yet their intention for being angry is not that they are obstinate or defiant. This is the time during which they need the most support, empathy, and encouragement.

Everything people with autism do is based on rules. While making their rules, they rationalize each step along the way. The rules may seem bizarre to the neurotypical. When the autie is asked to explain his thought processes, he often cannot. This is especially true if he has Obsessive Compulsive Disorder as a concomitant condition. An example of one of my rules is what I did to become the most productive person in my department when I worked as a Driver Trip Report clerk for Penske Truck Leasing. Being at my desk editing and typing reports all day was something I enjoyed doing. However, going along at the usual pace had me dead last in productivity in comparison with the other fifteen people in the department. It wasn't until I came up with my own set of rules as to *how* to type out the information in each column, and it wasn't until I invented my *own* coding system for the editing process that I soared. I made up steps my brain could comprehend to make a more proficient connection with the rest of me, that is my typing ability, my reading speed, etc. My rules not only made things easier for me to understand and organize but they also made them more entertaining and interesting. The changes were, however, quite annoying to my coworkers.

There were times that our supervisor would advise us about changes regarding how a certain state's travel permit should be handled or what extra information needed to be included for a specific leasing customer. While other people merely grumbled and adapted, I had to make a study of the change. I had to figure out where I could insert the new rules into my already-established routine to avoid confusion and to minimize any loss of proficiency. I struggled until I established new rules, and the change in routine eventually became an ingrained pattern. Although this is an example of a change in a way of doing things such as manual tasks, major change such as jobs themselves, losing a parent, or moving to another part of the country can be quite devastating. Whether small or large, changes can, and often do, cause mental wear and tear on the person with autism.

It is important for the parent, teacher, caretaker, health professional, and employer of someone with autism to keep in constant contact with them while they are going through a change. The National Autistic Society has some of the best words of advice I've seen regarding handling change in the

"Living With Autism" section of their website. The crisis one experiences while going through both large and small changes should never be belittled or taken lightly. It really is a big deal. As for me, I came to accept change, although not always welcoming it, after a significant period of spiritual development, thanks to my meditation routines. Once I started to see and experience the wonders of the Universe that lie beyond conscious comprehension while in deep states of meditation, I came to realize that everything is part of a bigger picture. Thusly, I am being *challenged* to change as I discover that the larger part of me, my consciousness itself, is the most important thing there is.

I talked previously about the process of the purification of samskaras whereby a person develops the natural inclination to let go of that which does not serve him. This is indeed the biggest and most beneficial change a person with autism may ever experience. On the other side of the kriyas lies a whole new world, one where strict adherence to rules no longer exists. Once my conscience was innately filled with a new sense of freedom, I associated my sense of self with something larger than merely what I do in life or the routines I have. Even though rulemaking still exists, routines became easier to change. After all, the autistic brain is hardwired for rulemaking. Changes became less of a burden, though, and in fact more beneficial for me to progress and evolve. Rules were no longer designed for the purpose of fulfilling someone else's wishes or for fitting an expectation as best as I could. They were intended to make me a more proficient servant to the Divine's purpose for me. This became the modus operandi of my entire being. It wasn't all about me anymore.

Before one reaches an "enlightened" way of incorporating change into their life, it is important to keep in mind the very first step: taking a deep breath. Breath itself gives the body and the mind their life force, or *prana*. Prana provides oxygen. Oxygen keeps us alive. When you have a well-oxygenated brain, you can think clearer and relax better. This is why monitoring your breathing is such an important part of any relaxation routine. Rational decisions and better choices come from a calm, clear mind. My word of advice that I tell fellow auties who are confronted by change is to have your outburst if you will. See it as a chance to vent. But then take a deep breath and get down to figuring out how the change will be dealt with.

What works best, ultimately, is seeing the situation objectively. Auties tend to look at things very subjectively; everything is happening *to* them. Objective vision comes from detachment. Detachment is automatically developed through meditation. It is a natural response to the realization of the bigger picture. You come to know that change is not only inevitable but that it is an imperative part of your own growth. It opens a new door to the development of your potentials. It opens doors to possibilities. It presents to you the next lesson in life that needs to be learned. Sometimes the change can take you in a negative direction that can be painful, certainly. That's where the term "growing pains" fits in nicely. But once a new routine has been added to the rules, you can relax a bit. You can relax in confidence, knowing that the next time you need to make a change, you have all the tools you need to handle it.

14

Regarding "Alternative" Medicine

The practice of Western medicine as we know it has been around for only about 150 years. To say that healing arts such as herbology, acupuncture, Reiki, and chiropractic are the "alternative" is a misnomer. One cannot replace the other. While it is true that western medicine has saved countless lives, thanks to medications and procedures that have been invented to save people whose lives are in danger, it has also caused much harm by creating false paradigms, as I pointed out earlier in this book. Since we've never seen a day in our lifetime when alternative medicine was mainstream, it is important for us to reconnect, so to speak, with what once was. First, we need to take a look at when and why the rift happened which separated the two schools of thought.

Throughout history, there has always been a swinging of the pendulum between the favoring of traditionally manufactured medications and holistic remedies. Even after the American Medical Association (AMA) was formed in 1847, herbal concoctions were preferred over pharmaceutical agents. About this time, surgical procedures were being popularized by the invention of anesthetics. It wasn't until the 1870s that medical schools finally established criteria of what should be taught in their curricula. It was also when states started forming medical licensing boards. This is not to say that medicine didn't already have its share of advances, as it was quite progressive in Europe and around the world. However, the AMA was the first professional organization formed to regulate its practice. By the 1870s, the AMA had deemed it more profitable for American doctors to use only drugs made by pharmaceutical companies. It then declared anything else to be unsafe because they were considered based on belief and not science. This declaration also put the newly-created profession of osteopathy in the same "unscientific" category.

When chiropractic came along in 1895, the AMA acted swiftly to try to quash this bold new healing art, science, and philosophy of wellness. Throughout the early 1900s, chiropractors throughout the U.S. were being thrown in jail for "practicing medicine without a license." This was despite the fact that chiropractic schools could be found everywhere and states were forming their own regulatory chiropractic boards. In late 1963, the AMA stepped up its efforts to contain and eliminate the chiropractic profession by forming the Committee on Quackery. They were quite confident of their witch hunt after it successfully overtook and eliminated osteopathy as it was known and practiced in 1962. It wasn't until 1976 when chiropractors started to fight back. With chiropractors now being licensed and a gaining popularity in all 50 states as of 1974, it was time for the tide to turn. A group of five chiropractors from Chicago headed up by Dr. Chester Wilk brought an antitrust lawsuit against the AMA and at least four of its ally organizations. Eleven years later, on September 25, 1987, U.S. District Court judge Susan Getzendanner ruled that the AMA was indeed guilty of its efforts after countless studies and testimonials were presented proving chiropractic's efficacy and superiority. That's when the chiropractic profession finally started to gain the credibility and respect it deserved, 92 years after it was founded.

Naturopathic physicians have the same uphill fight to gain status. Beginning as the *Natural Cure Movement of Europe* in the 19th century, it was first called "naturopathy" in 1895. Between 1901 and 1930, this nature-based healing art became widely accepted, and 25 states recognized it as a profession. But that all changed after the AMA's successful smear campaign against varying healing systems, that is anything that was not created by itself. As the pendulum started to swing back toward natural healing during the 1970s, naturopathy once again stepped into view. Nowadays, there are seven schools of naturopathic medicine and only nineteen states that license Naturopathic Doctors (NDs) as primary care professionals.

Because of the AMA's efforts to hide these healing arts, all in the name of profit and egoism, most of the American public has no idea what other options exist other than the ones they are told about by the Western medical system. In its eyes, Western medicine is all that exists. However, they are starting to come around since more people of status, such as the Dalai Lama, are making a push for their acceptance as well as a more compassionate approach to patient care. Yes, a compassionate, patient-centered approach is certainly something which became lost in all the science, ego, and technological advances.

In order to make the much-needed shift in focus, many hospitals are now creating departments that offer Complementary and Alternative Medicine (CAM) therapies, some which include chiropractic care. The Cleveland Clinic hospital in Cleveland, Ohio is one such place. The Cleveland Clinic has become a pioneer in the study and acceptance of Reiki healing in particular. Thanks to the National Center for Complementary & Alternative Medicine, a subdivision of the U.S. Department of Health and Human Services, more research is being funded and the results published on the myriad of alternative healing arts. The NCCAM also keeps a database of the various named healing arts and a synopsis of their philosophies and methodologies. Let's take a look at some of the studies on alternative medicine that have been done to date:

- Reed, W.R., et al. "Chiropractic Management of Primary Nocturnal Enuresis". *Journal of Manipulative and Physiological Therapeutics*. Dec. 1993. Vol. 17, Iss. 9, pp. 596-600. Elsevier B.V. Web. Feb. 15, 2015

Forty-six children with an active history of nighttime bed wetting were studied to examine the efficacy of chiropractic adjustments in relieving their condition. After ten weeks of care, thirteen of the thirty-one participants in the treatment group experienced at least a 50% reduction in their symptoms compared to the fifteen in the control group which experienced no change.

- Tuchin, Peter, J., et al. "A randomized controlled trial of chiropractic spinal manipulative therapy for migraine". *Journal of Manipulative and Physiological Therapeutics*. Feb. 2000. Vol. 23, Iss. 2, pp. 91-95. Elsevier B.V. Web. Feb. 15, 2015.

120 people participated in this study in which sixteen spinal adjustments were administered over the course of two months. The average outcome among the eighty-three people in the treatment group showed that there was a significant improvement in the participants' condition. 22% said that there was a 90% reduction in their migraine

occurrences while another 50% reported a significant improvement in the severity of their episodes.

- Berman, Brian, M., et al. "Effectiveness of Acupuncture as Adjunctive Therapy in Osteoarthritis of the Knee". *Annals of Internal Medicine*. Dec. 21, 2004. Vol. 141, No. 12, pp. 901-910. American College of Physicians. Web. Feb. 16, 2015

570 subjects age 50 or older who had chronic pain from osteoarthritis of the knee participated in this study. Of the 140 participants in the treatment group who actually completed the entire treatment regimen of 23 acupuncture treatments over the course of 26 weeks, a significant improvement was reported in their level of function after only 8 weeks. A significant improvement in their level of pain was noted after the 26th week.

- Melchert, Dieter, et al. "Acupuncture in patients with tension-type headache: randomised controlled trial". *British Medical Journal*. Aug. 11, 2005. Vol. 331, Iss. 7513, pp. 376-382. BMJ Publishing Group, Ltd. Web. Feb. 16, 2015

270 people participated in this 26-week study to see if acupuncture was effective in the treatment of chronic tension headaches. 132 received acupuncture treatments and another 63 received acupuncture for conditions other than the headaches. 75 were placed on a waiting list, and they entered the study after the 12th week. What was surprising was that all three groups received positive results. 46% in the acupuncture group, 35% in the "other" group, and 4% in the "waiting list" group reported a 50% reduction in the

occurrence of their headaches.

- Speca, Michael, et al. "A Randomized, Wait-List Controlled Clinical Trial: The Effect of a Mindfulness Meditation-Based Stress Reduction Program on Mood and Symptoms of Stress in Cancer Outpatients". *Psychosomatic Medicine*. Sept./Oct. 2000. Vol. 62, Iss. 5, pp. 613-622. Wolters Kluwer. Web. Feb. 20, 2015

Ninety subjects with varying types and stages of cancer took part in this study. The treatment group took part in weekly meditation sessions lasting ninety minutes each for seven weeks with additional home meditation exercises. At the end of the study, the participants showed significantly lower stress levels and better mood control than the control group subjects. 65% reported a reduction in mood disturbance while 31% experienced a reduction in symptoms of stress.

- Sudsuang, Ratree, et all. "Effect of Buddhist meditation on serum cortisol and total protein levels, blood pressure, pulse rate, lung volume and reaction time". *Physiology & Behavior*. September 1991. Vol. 50, Iss. 3, pp. 543-548. Elsevier B.V. Web. Feb. 20, 2015

This study was done using Dhammakaya Buddhist meditation, a non-traditional method which teaches that the *nirvana* experience is actually the attainment of the state of the "true Self." Fifty-two males were studied using this type of meditation, and they were compared to a control group of thirty males. After meditation sessions, blood levels of the test subjects were checked. A significant reduction in cortisol, one of the main hormones produced during stress responses, was noted along with a significant reduction in blood pressure.

These are just a very few of the many studies done on just a very few of the many alternative medicine healing arts. Most of these practices originated hundreds, perhaps thousands, of years ago. One of the first books ever written on the subject of yoga was the *Yoga Sutras of Patanjali* circa 400 A.D. Buddhism began about 580 B.C. The origins of Chinese acupuncture date back roughly 4,000 years. Ancient Greek and Chinese literature and Egyptian hieroglyphs indicate the use of early forms of chiropractic care to treat diseases and disorders. People who are more in-tune with these practices are celebrating their reemergence after years of oppression and attempted abolition.

Because of the lies being fed to people by the medical establishment, much of what people *think* they know about these healing arts is an extremely narrow view of what they actually are. For example, most people believe that chiropractic is a last-resort treatment for low back pain. In reality, it is the premier method, separate and independent of any medical paradigm, of optimizing the body's overall functionality. Because of chiropractic's ability to restore normal nervous system function via the realignment of the skeletal frame, people have been able to overcome a myriad of various illnesses and conditions, of which low back pain is a mere blip on the radar. Likewise, massage is so much more than just a relaxing feel-good luxury, and Reiki and acupuncture are not just de-stressing methods. There is so much that the person who wants to know about them can learn and experience for themselves if they just see past the blind judgments that had been fed to them by the medical establishment or by closed-minded people who have no education regarding them.

The Western medical system has lots to learn from the formally-trained practitioners of these much-older, time-tested healing arts. First and foremost, they can learn that the people they are treating are living, breathing human beings with names, lives, families, hopes, and dreams. This is the way of thinking that the legendary Hunter "Patch" Adams, M.D. wanted to integrate into modern medical education. Likewise, holistic healing practitioners need to do what they do from their center, a heart filled with sincerity. Most do. But there are those who need to quell their *own* egos. They need to realize that the Western medicine practices may be what ends up saving them if they are ever faced with a life-or-death crisis. As I pointed out in the beginning of this chapter, Western medicine and alternative medicine are each separate and distinct. One cannot replace the other. When used *in conjunction* with each other, even the toughest of health challenges can be improved significantly.

15

Mainstreaming Autism

If there's one situation worthy of a complete paradigm shift, it's how people on the autism spectrum are treated by neurotypicals. In order for auties to be treated as equals, only *one* bit of effort is required on the part of the neurotypical, and that is the acceptance of the fact that their view of the world will be changed. It is a much-needed change. The unique viewpoint of the autie can often add the missing piece of the puzzle when trying to solve problems, form better solutions, find better ways of doing something, and arriving at a conclusion more proficiently. Different autistic brains process information in different ways. One person on the spectrum may envision pictures, as I do. Another may form musical patterns. Yet another will think mathematically. Any one of these coupled with the neurotypical's way of thinking can paint a unique picture of mastery that is indeed celebrated. Thus, it is actually *vital* for people with ASD to be included on any team or workforce for success to be swift and imminent.

Mainstreaming works best when one other member of the team or teaching staff is designated as the mentor to the person with autism. He/she needs to be familiar with the autistic person's ways of thinking and communicating, habits, stress capacity, stimming or outburst tendencies, etc. Even if it means that the autie prefers to work alone in his ventures *at first*, the mentor needs to give him the space and time he needs. There almost always *will* come a time when the person with autism figures his way around to the point where he is very much an integral and important part of the team. These same rules apply when a child with ASD is placed in a typical classroom. As long as he is allowed to produce results in a timely manner using his own means of problem-solving, even if such methods appear to the teacher to be disruptive or incongruent with the normal schedule, he must be allowed to proceed. The mentor is, therefore, the ambassador of the words once spoken by the famous ventriloquist and education consultant Ignacio "Nacho" Estrada, "If a child can't learn the way we teach, maybe we should teach the way they learn."

Now the comments may flow forth from the naysayers, "That autistic guy is slowing us down." Goodness knows how many times I've been accused of holding up the process, often being let go from jobs because I was too slow. That was a long long time before I ever knew I had autism. For those positions and learning situations in which I excelled, I did so because I had that (unbeknownst) mentor while continuing to be a part of the team. The mentors didn't tell me *how* to do my work. They were merely there to give me every chance I needed to figure it out for myself. My learning process was, and still is, heavily dependent on thinking in pictures, whether I was memorizing a piece of music, multitasking several critical tasks on an ambulance crew, or learning how to operate a new therapy machine or respiratory ventilator. Once I excelled and became an integral part of the work team, my capacity for critical analysis and decision making was right on par with the most experienced of the bunch.

Other words of discouragement may follow. "How much will it cost to dedicate one person to be a mentor to the autistic ones?" Well, first of all, a question like that means that a paradigm shift has not yet been made. You'll never be able to accomplish this without one. This is why I see "autistic specialist" programs fail. There's nobody there that knows enough about autism, there's not enough money invested to support the program, and the program is being used as a dumping tank for problem kids, most of whom don't even have an official autism spectrum disorder diagnosis. For a mainstreamed mentorship program to work, whether in a school or in a work setting, it would be best to consult with someone who actually *has* autism, who knows how the autistic brain functions, who is also educated and knows about leadership and management styles. *That* is a *real* autism expert. Once the points in this paragraph are digested and assimilated, a successful program can then be put in place.

There is yet another paradigm shift that needs to be made. The Johns Hopkins School of Education explains, "No one program or strategy will benefit all students, ASD or not. Any program utilized by a school system will only be as effective as the educators in charge of implementing it. They must, therefore, be afforded as much training as needed and the support of their administration[56]." Therefore, the idea of mainstreaming, or inclusion as it is more recently referred to, must take into account the learning needs of everyone *subjectively*. I frequently hear complaints about the objective system that becomes a problem for the unique non-autistic individual, a system which often leads the parents to make the decision to homeschool their child if he or she can't be placed in a gifted program. In the workplace, the same consideration must be given to the freethinking adult whose creativity and individuality need to be nurtured. To add to that, the administration must be on par with, completely supportive of, and in congruence with the goals and operations of an inclusion program.

In a study published in the February 2014 issue of International Journal of Inclusive Education, Sally Lindsay et al. outlines five components to successfully integrating children with autism into a mainstream classroom:

a.) Advocating for resources, such as educational supports and assistive technologies, and essential training in how to work with children with ASDs,

b.) Tailored teaching methods focusing more on the delivery method rather than the content,

c.) Teamwork between all staff, teachers, assistants, and therapists involved in the creation of effective teaching strategies,

d.) Building a rapport with the parents and students, and

e.) Building a climate of acceptance in the classroom by minimizing opportunity for exclusion and increasing disability awareness.[57]

In the same study, Lindsay points out that including a person with an ASD in the group or classrooms gives others the opportunity to learn more about the challenges of autism.

There are some schools and private groups that are breaking the mold by enrolling children with high-functioning autism in various programs to help them integrate. Programs such as Vanderbilt University's SENSE Theater Camp, the Social Competence Intervention Program, and other drama-based programs are showing much promise in helping older children learn body language and appropriate communication skills so they don't feel so clueless among their peers. Drama classes allow for the comfort of role playing in controlled and guided situations whereby children are allowed to act out real-life situations and learn the appropriate responses without judgment. These programs are run by trained drama therapists, and they make use of peer models. Above all else, the schools that utilize such programs celebrate the neurological diversity of their students because important tools, such as patience, are learned by everyone.[58]

I feel that such an inclusion program is quite possible to manage in any work setting, just as it is at these schools, should a company decide to create a truly equal opportunity environment while focusing on the preservation of basic human rights. From personal experience, I can assure you that cliquish people will be the first to bully and gossip, and they will want no part of interacting with anyone who challenges their narrow and condescending mindsets. Therefore, building a climate of acceptance is a crucial step to making any inclusion program successful. This is not always easy to come by when a company supervisor is just as obstinate, as I have observed over the years. Nobody likes having to deal with someone who is seen as "different." Mainstreaming can only succeed in an environment that is willing to accept it.

I was pleasantly surprised to discover how much information has been written in recent times on the very topic of mainstreaming, especially about the creation of various inclusion program training resources. No school or company should be at a loss when it comes to being able to provide equal opportunity to people (yes, living, breathing, thinking *people* who have feelings, ideas, hopes. dreams. and lives) with Autism Spectrum Disorder. It's not about seeing the "different" people as equals. It's about completely annihilating the notion of difference altogether. It's not about perking up to pay special attention to someone who is perceived as "less than." It's about throwing away the idea that there is a lesser or greater. Equal means *equal*, as in 1+1=2. 1+1 is neither greater than nor less than 2. Nor is it *different* than 2. It *is* 2.

Thanks to an organization that came into being in 2010 called Think Beyond the Label, the inclusion of people with all sorts of disabilities and differences in the workforce became a lot easier. TBTL offers a host of resources to help employers make the mainstreaming process smoother. They also offer job listings for those seeking employment. Mainstreaming is not about doing away with diagnoses and labels. It is about knowing that everyone is on par and has something to offer *despite* their condition. In fact, one's unique perspective is inherent *because* of their condition, which in turn makes the bigger picture more complete. Completeness is what adds strength to the work force and to the learning environment. Completeness means that everybody's view is taken into account and given equal consideration in the learning/decision-making process. Inclusion, mainstreaming, equal opportunity, is not about trying to obtain a manageable median. It is about adding more color to the canvas.

16

The Avadhuta State

There is a type of human being who is surely in this world but not of it. They have completed their spiritual journey, their liberation process, that commenced the day their Kundalini energy was awakened. Such a person is known as a *Siddha*. The 2015 Collins English Dictionary defines a Siddha as "A person who has achieved perfection; a saint." "Perfection" refers to living in a completely ego-free state, un-influenced by worldly matters yet completely aware of and involved with the world. Such saints walk among us. There have been many Siddhas throughout the ages, and there will continue to be many in the ages to come. Some are gurus who have devotees and disciples. Others are humble and nameless creatures who may appear to be lost souls. The important thing to know is that they are here for a specific purpose. Their presence in this world brings balance to the powers in the Universe. They maintain the dynamics of the dualistic natures of yin and yang.

In rare instances, a Siddha is found in this world who is beyond all worldly comprehension. Usually, such a person is born a Siddha, not made into one through ascetic practices. This person is known as an *avadhuta*. If an avadhuta were to be found wandering the streets in the U.S. or any developed country today, it wouldn't be long before he was carted off to a mental institution. They have no concept of customs or laws, and some may not feel the need to wear clothing. They may live in garbage dumps, rarely speak, and might possess powers that defy logic. The reason for such extremely odd behavior is because their state of awareness lies completely and continuously in the bliss of divine experience. The concept of an avadhuta is surely a difficult one to grasp. What brings it all down to Earth is reading the life stories of famous avadhutas such as Bhagawan Nityananda of Kanhangadh and Ganeshpuri, Zipruanna of Nasirabad, and Saint Dnyaneshwar. In between their states of oblivion to the world around them, they interacted with others, they traveled, they wrote, and they taught. But because of their extreme strangeness, they could never exist in a modern society.

It is one thing to know that you are in this world to accomplish something, even when a Siddha. It is another to dwell constantly in a state of cosmic bliss, completely immersed in and undivided from Universal Consciousness, as is an avadhuta. Their presence signifies the dire need for balance in the world when yin energy, that which is dark and negative, starts to become too strong. The question may arise as to why one would *want* to be in such a state. Is it an escape from the world? Is it a sign of laziness? Of indolence? Along with these questions, the difference between a genuine avadhuta and an escapist who wants to elude his life must be explained. That can be easily determined by their intent. One intends to have no interests, and the other is overwhelmed, lovingly so, with everything.

To add a bit of concreteness to what the avadhuta state looks like, let's turn the topic to a five-minute segment of Craig McCracken's cartoon *Wander Over Yonder* in the episode "The Funk." In an attempt to help the villain Lord Hater break out of his funk, his minion, Commander Peepers, introduces him to a race of rather hollow and otiose beings known as Mooplexians. The Mooplexians appeared weak and insignificant, and Lord Hater could easily taunt them and kick them around, literally. This amused Lord Hater, and it made him feel superior to the point where he felt like his usual malicious self once again. But, in the end, all that the humiliating funnery did was pull the Mooplexians' consciousnesses back into their bodies in order to give Lord Hater a verbal thrashing along with a rather Siddha-like explanation of where their awareness goes when it is not present within the physical body. Much like the Mooplexians, an avadhuta can appear to be an empty shell that merely breathes, while, in reality, he is enjoying the inner Play of Consciousness. As a result, he is often shunned or taunted by the small-minded who have no concept of spiritual evolution.

Unfortunately, the type of bullying Lord Hater unleashed occurs quite often to those whose minds are elsewhere. People on the autism spectrum, INFJs, daydreamers, and avadhuta all have that in common. In typically less-cultured places such as India, one may throw rocks at or shoo away the unwelcome or disruptive avadhuta. Here in the U.S., such people with the wondrous, bright minds but yet quiet or spacy demeanors are oftentimes the victims of unwarranted and unjust discrimination. Whether physically harming or not, such actions are indeed bullying in various forms. It is *imperative* for schools and employers to address the issue of bullying by initiating anti-bullying programs. Programs such as those created by PACER Center, Inc. are great tools to implement. It is equally as vital for the one being bullied to maintain his sense of dignity, uniqueness, and his right to roam within the inner depths that make him who he is. This is made easier when the individual realizes that bullying is actually caused by fear, which is, in reality, an acknowledgment of the bully's own insecurity.

Just as with avadhuta, nonverbal people with autism are "in their own world." But their world is far from limited. It is big, *very* big. The *inner* dialog, the creativity, the inspiration, the visualization of and interaction with other worlds, the coming and going into and out of dreamlike states, the roaming of the Universe within, the unrelenting flow of mystical bliss —— it is all part of being in that state that only an avadhuta, and also an inwardly-aware autie, can enjoy. When the enlightened avadhuta finally does emerge to interact with the physical world around him, his words bring people to their knees. They are never spoken without reason or intent. Likewise, the person with autism who has spent a great deal of his or her life immersed in that divine oblivion will eventually turn their attention and actions outward to serve the world around them. It happens when it is time, at a time when they figure out just *how* to be in it.

Most of us will never meet a Siddha in our lifetime, unless we actually become one that is. I am quite certain that none of us will ever encounter an avadhuta. We all have the ability to approach the state of a Siddha simply by making a regular practice of meditating. For the person with autism, forms of yoga which focus on controlling the breath, placing the body in specific positions, and the development of concentration abilities show promising results in helping him or her manage their difficult behaviors and anxiety levels[59]. But I propose taking it to the next level. That means focusing on growing in a spiritual way through transcendence and detachment as opposed to merely resolving problematic issues.

Yoga is the best practice for reaching the goal of spiritual enlightenment. The word "yoga," though, is merely a general term just as the word "medicine" doesn't specify which treatment will help a certain condition. A specific type of yoga should be selected and stuck to. It is by adhering to a philosophy and routine and not jumping from one to the other that we progress. The various poses, the method of breathing, the straightening of the posture, the inward focus, are all intrinsic to various types of yoga, and they all have one and the same purpose: to guide and direct the Kundalini energy. Spiritual enlightenment is the end product of this process. It is the culmination of Kundalini's journey. This is what makes a Siddha.

The literal meaning of the word *yoga* is "union with the Supreme Being" in the Hindi language. For an avadhuta, yoga is a constant *state of being*. The avadhuta is absorbed in this union so completely that everything else is trivial, even his own physical existence. An avadhuta is a Siddha who is literally an embodiment of God Consciousness, existing at a particular point in time to bring balance to the world and to awaken others. Otherwise, their karmic destiny is complete. They have reached the ultimate pitch of energy vibration. Because of that, they are free to come and go at will with their consciousness as well as with their life force energy. Their presence is completely up to them.

17

The End of the Funk

I had a feeling that 2015 would be a good year. Both Becky and I had struggled financially since the day we met. Without help from Becky's family, we may have ended up homeless together. Such a struggle was Becky's way of life for only a few short years. For me, it existed for most of my adult life. Soon after we started living together, Becky endured interview after interview in search of gainful employment in her profession as a social worker. I was making list after list of different types of establishments to which I would advertise both my ministerial services and my holistic healing practice. Neither one of us received much in the way of a glimmer of hope. In mid-January, though, things suddenly changed for both of us.

It started first for Becky when she finally found work in her field as a counselor for people with various psychological disorders. Her struggle was finally over after having lost a previous job doing the same thing almost three years earlier. As for me, I was still contacting places on my lists. This time, I was focusing on fitness centers. Out of the forty-one places I advertised to, all of which were located within twenty-two miles of where we lived, only one responded. Its response was positive. The owner of a fitness center located in the village of Temple was excited to have me work there. He had a chiropractor in his fitness center who left two years earlier to open an office elsewhere. He was hoping for someone else to come along ever since. But that left me with both a dilemma and an incentive. I wasn't telling people I practiced chiropractic since I didn't hold a current license. I was, instead, advertising my licensure-exempt services. Because of this new interest, this new light, I suddenly had the push I needed to get my license back.

While the picture was looking more promising, the obstacles that I was suddenly met with weren't so easy to deal with. The main reason why I never attempted to renew my Pennsylvania license when I came back was because I simply gave up. Years of trying to get a practice going with no success at all finally took its toll. Yes, I served some people well along the way. But I was never able to make a living at it. Now, for the first time since returning to Pennsylvania, somebody was showing exceptional interest in what I had to offer. It wasn't a paying job, but being located in a fitness center seemed like an ideal opportunity. The second reason why I never renewed my license was now a bigger issue than before — the fact that I would have to ask my brother for money to do so since he had control over my inheritance coupled with the expectation of "no" for an answer. The $3K allotment was all I could be given in a year, and the rest of the money in the trust was for emergency use only. Now I *had* to ask. I was pleasantly surprised and relieved, though, when my brother said "yes."

It seemed that everything was underway, and I prepared my application. I sent it off to the state as quickly as I could. I told the owner of the fitness center to be patient while I "upgrade" my services to be more marketable and more capable of helping his members. Although that was okay with him, two more roadblocks eventually presented themselves. For one, he told me a couple things that didn't sit too well with me. First of all, I wouldn't be allowed to post signage of my presence or to solicit the members of the fitness center. It seemed counterproductive to the whole reason for me being there in the first place. However, with the offer of an amazingly low by-the-hour rental rate, I wasn't going to pull out. In addition to the owner's restrictions, I also wouldn't be allowed to simply be there to await walk-in clients. Everything had to be scheduled in advance.

The other roadblock I ran into had to do with Pennsylvania's relicensing rules. Since I hadn't been licensed in PA since 2002, and because I didn't have a currently-active license anywhere, the state board wanted me to take the Special Purposes Examination for Chiropractic. The SPEC exam would require me to study everything I ever learned in school about orthopedic and neurological diagnoses. Also, the exam costs $1,500. I felt that my quest to renew my license had come to an unfortunate and disheartening end since I had no intention on wracking my brain due to some lame rule. The other option, which I was also not a fan of, was for me to obtain a license in another state and practice in that state for a minimum of twenty months.

During the time in which I was hopeful and positive, an inspiration had hit me from out of the blue. I flashed back to the time I had a practice at the former Pocono Plaza Truck Stop in Bartonsville between September 2001 and June 2002. Half of all my business was from commercial motor vehicle drivers who were in need of their biennial Driver Fitness Determination Examination, otherwise known as the "D.O.T. physical." I mentioned to the owner of the fitness center that I could become certified to provide these physicals as part of my services. After all, the center was located along a major U.S. highway, and there was much industry in the area whereby such a service would be needed. When I practiced at the truck stop all those years ago, certification to provide these exams was not necessary, other than having a current license to practice, of course. Now, examiners needed to go through a training program with the U.S. Department of Transportation and become certified as Medical Examiner in order to do these physicals. Once examiners are certified, their names are placed on a national registry list so people can find them. Since this program was less than a year old at that point, I figured I could get in on it early before the market became saturated, and people would find me simply because I'd be one of just a few on the list. "What a great way to build a practice for someone who is terribly introverted," I thought. Being a Nationally Registered Certified Medical Examiner (NRCME) then became the main focus of my license renewal effort.

But with the obstacles to renewing my Pennsylvania license in front of me, I sunk down a bit. I figured the Universe was telling me I should probably follow Rule #6 of my own Spiritual Laws of Success. Maybe being a "doctor" wasn't what I was supposed to be doing in life. Perhaps I should be focused more on the services I provide as an Ordained Minister. After all, I can still do spiritual healing work, taking care of the body, mind, and spirit holistically. Maybe this was all part of my own evolution, the guiding toward my true calling? During this time, I changed my National Provider Identifier type from a chiropractor to one who offers non-medical religious services and pastoral counseling. I was done with the whole health care thing, finally, after thirty-two years.

Almost two months went by. Then, out of the blue, inspiration and a driving force hit me even harder than before. The message going around inside my head was, "I didn't come all this way to simply give up. I am certainly capable of more!" And with that, I decided to take the twenty-month-in-another-state option, and I applied for a new license in the next closest state, New Jersey. After all, New Jersey didn't have the ridiculous rules that Pennsylvania did. I explained the situation to my brother, and once again he allowed me to have the money I needed. Away I was again, hoping for a positive word and eventual entrance into the NRCME program. In less than half the time it took me to receive a negative reply from the PA Board of Chiropractic, I received my license to practice in New Jersey. Seven days after that, I enrolled in the Department of Transportation's Certified Medical Examiner program.

This whole ordeal taught me an important lesson. It's not just about not giving up or about needing a sense of purpose. It's about listening to your gut instinct and following your heart's beckoning. There will be that battle between the head and the heart which will make you go back and forth. In the end, you will *always* do the right thing if you listen to your heart. If being a doctor was not what I was supposed to be doing, I would have never received such a push from the inside to keep going. You will know for certain you are doing the right thing when that inner voice talks. The Upanishads repeatedly refer to the heart as the seat of God. As Joel Osteen always says, "God spoke to me — not out loud, but in a feeling I got right here (as he holds his hand over his solar plexus)." That really is how God communicates with us. It's just up to us to recognize that this is divine inspiration, our connectedness to our Source, at work.

Although becoming licensed again and being certified as a D.O.T. Medical Examiner didn't end the struggle all at once, it did open a huge door. I passed my certification exam and was then listed on the D.O.T.'s website on June 2. After that, I contacted several truck stops in northern New Jersey to see if any of them would allow me to set up an office there, just like the one I had thirteen years earlier in the Poconos. Only one was interested, and it wasn't even a full-service truck stop. As for the rest, they were not only uninterested but they were rather arrogantly against the idea. It was a good thing, that the one that was interested was located just across the river from the Pennsylvania state line in Phillipsburg. This was the ideal location for me to meet with and take care of patients from both states. I also figured that I could do house calls as well with my minivan, so I listed myself in several zip codes throughout northern New Jersey, 265 of them in all. From then on, I received several calls each week from people needing D.O.T. physicals.

Over the course of the next year, my income level increased dramatically to the point where I could finally say goodbye to the days of living below the poverty line. I converted the back of my minivan into an actual office that people could fit inside since I found myself traveling throughout northern New Jersey quite a bit. Visiting people at their homes, receiving calls from companies needing physicals for their fleet of drivers, and meeting people at the truck stop in Phillipsburg became a weekly routine. In April 2016, I enjoyed my busiest and most profitable month in my life when I performed 42 D.O.T. physicals and made more than $4,200, including the income from a surge of structural alignment and Reiki clients in Pennsylvania. It was good to *finally* feel as though I was making a living at doing what I was meant to do in life.

Because both our financial situations had improved, Becky and I moved into a new house, our *own* house, in

December of 2015. It was bought by her stepdad Ken, and the plan was for us to pay him the monthly mortgage. The house was an older home, built in 1951, and it still contained almost all the original cabinetry and appliances. Bordering with both a scenic golf course and a major state highway, it seemed the ideal location. The most affluent part was that the property was zoned commercial. Because we had a spacious loft above the garage, the wheels in our heads started turning. We both desired to eventually have our own offices, and we also had visions of creating a place for spiritual camaraderie. Slowly but surely, we started converting the loft into the place that we had envisioned. We finally had the money to do things, and we got right down to making some of our life goals a reality.

18

Self-Advocacy

For a person to be able to stand up for themselves in the real world, they must approach it from the angle of equality. This is a non-issue for the neurotypical, outgoing, worldly person. But for a person with ASD, an introvert, a victim of bullying, or someone who simply has a different way of being, it is a very real and disheartening struggle. Remember that you're not trying to prove yourself to someone, not even to anyone. You're not showing a potential employer that you're down and trying to get up again. Self-advocacy is about *already* being in the position of authority and being comfortable where you are in life. If a person does not respond in kind or reacts in a condescending way, there really is no point in wanting to be associated with them. This rule applies whether it is an individual or a group. In that case, you really aren't losing anything. You merely weed out your own garden and move on.

Many people on the autism spectrum feel overwhelmed with the world around them. If they aren't very proficient at social skills, they might feel powerless when stating their position in it. They might even come across as overbearing because of an underlying aura of insecurity. Even if this is the situation, a person with autism who wants to be self-sufficient can be successful. Inside each and every person who needs encouraging and support lies the one who can give it to them. This is demonstrated in a variety of situations by Dr. David D. Burns in his book "Feeling Good: The New Mood Therapy." Whether it be discovering ways to boost one's self-esteem, dealing with dysfunctional thoughts including guilt, developing a new perspective, or coping with hostility, one can change the way he feels about and interact with their environment. This is accomplished by writing down one's existing perspective, identifying the problem with it, and then coming up with a more rational response. It is so empowering when a person realizes that they really *are* in control of their own destiny.

Because Dr. Burns' methods may take some doing even for the non-autistic person, it's no wonder why the person who has difficulty navigating the social nuances of the world might feel clueless when attempting to be his own advocate. After all, autism is a different way of processing and interpreting information. Everything the autistic person experiences is scrutinized using the set of rules by which he navigates and by the black-and-white lens through which he views the world. This can lead to him digging his own holes that he can't seem to get out of. Therefore, the process of writing, identifying, and rationalizing becomes one of setting new rules and finding the shades of gray in between. The more masterful a person on the autism spectrum becomes at this, the more likely he is to gain the confidence and the stamina that is vital to being his own advocate.

If a person is truly unsure of where his strengths lie and of what they need to be doing in life, they need not look any further than to Tom Rath's Clifton StrengthsFinder. StrengthsFinder is not a fly-by-night quiz that one can find on social media. It is a self-assessment tool that was developed by Dr. Donald O. Clifton, the father of Strengths Psychology. It was first published in 1998 by Gallup Press, and an update followed in 2007. To date, it has helped millions of people discover their areas of strength and how they can capitalize on them.[60] This is of paramount importance to the person on that autism spectrum whose focus *must* be on the developing of his strengths as opposed to the strengthening of his weaknesses. He may be physically unable to change a weakness simply because of the way his brain is hardwired or due to the way his physical body has developed. To focus on weaknesses assures years of frustration and a constant feeling of inadequacy.

The overall best way for someone to become their own advocate is to have a mentor who believes in them. I discussed the importance of mentors earlier in this book, and I cannot emphasize their vitalness enough. If not for my two greatest mentors, Larry Pisano, whose guidance led me to where I am professionally, and Betty McKeon, whose insight brought me to the spiritual height I enjoy, I have no idea where I'd be today. I am quite sure I wouldn't be writing this book. Finding my place in this world would have certainly taken me in a completely different direction. Despite my life having been fraught with disappointment, constant struggle, and a seemingly-continuous uphill battle, all ended up okay eventually, thanks to my ASD diagnosis. And because of years of dedication to building upon my strengths in one area, as opposed to trying to change a weakness, I am able to advocate for myself. I do so because of the confidence I have in my own abilities and my education, knowledge, and insight in those few areas in which I immersed myself. This is the approach the person on the autism spectrum must take if they wish to be successful with being their own hero.

19

Connections

The reason why any of us are here in this physical world is so we can connect — connect with others, connect with nature, connect with ourselves, and connect with our purpose. Most people do these things through outward interaction. Some do not have the innate ability to do this, so their method of connecting is aut (self, within)-istic in nature. Whether through autistic means or typical, one cannot escape the reality of the connectedness of everything. Nothing and nobody is separate from anything or anyone else. Just because of the very fact that we exist, this is true. Because of our connection, communication is constant. We are continuously communicating, whether verbally or not, and the energy of that communication speaks a lot louder than the physical act of doing so.

Earlier in this book, I talked about the concept of chi. Chi is a universal energy. It is omnipresent, ever-flowing, and intelligent. It *is* consciousness itself. It is the means by which the connectedness of everything exists. It is also the means by which all that is connected communicates. With typical communication, there is verbal or written interaction. But communication begins well before anything is ever said or written. It begins with intent, and that intent can be *felt* by people. This is evident when you get a certain vibe about a person, whether good or bad. Because communication is always a two-way street, one's *intent* is what attracts the right situations and the right people into one's life. It cannot be any other way. But because of both "lag time" and karma, results are not always imminent. Communication of an intent that is earnest, therefore, must be persistent.

People who are intuitive can perceive the movement of chi very well. It helps them discover hidden agenda, true intents, when and where healing may be needed, and it helps them to see the elephant in the room that needs tending to. Such people are often mistaken for being "psychic" or are praised for being insightful. In reality, they are merely being their observant selves. Anyone who tunes in and transcends above and beyond the purely physical, i.e. that which is merely seen and heard, can feel the movement of chi and know where it is going. It's not an otherworldly gift. It is the sixth sense that is so very keen in children, yet a vital part of our experience that tends to go away as we are taught to rely more on the concrete.

Now that we know more about this connection, we can look at it on a more global scale. Social media has certainly made the world a lot smaller. Because of this, the flocks of birds of a common feather have skyrocketed in size. Because of this, relationships can be created or destroyed, political careers made or broken, knowledge disseminated or discredited. Both legal and illegal activities have their forums. Crimes can be committed and prevented all through technology's creation of abundant connections. Thanks to this outlet, to this opportunity for chi to flow like never before, the door has been opened for paradigms to shift. We no longer need to live in the dark or do conventional things merely because "we've always done it that way." We have the opportunity to be educated, to gain knowledge, to make more informed decisions, and to create change. We no longer have to live in Plato's cave.

Whether talking about connection to our immediate surroundings or to people and causes around the globe, we have the ability to choose for ourselves how we are going to connect. We have the power to determine how chi will move from our own intent; each one of us *individually* is the consciousness that shifts paradigms. The question is who will be the hundredth monkey, and when will that permanent change take place? I feel it is closer than any of us realize. As far as us taking control of our own health care goes, more power is being grasped and decisions being made by the proactive society and less by the authoritative establishment since the early 1990s. With autism, we are starting to see the transition as more and more employers focus on hiring people with ASDs *because* of their giftedness. Spiritually, we cannot say when a major shift will take place. But because Earth is a dualistic world, there will always be battles between opposites. Some New-Agers, however, claim that the shift already took place on March 21, 2012, the dawning of the Age of Aquarius.

When one approaches the state of a living saint, giving up all attachment to beliefs, arguments, outcomes, and judgments, chi moves in a very different way and for a very different purpose. Through meditation, its purpose becomes the purifying of the mind and the liberation from the illusions of the world. How often do I hear people say, "When I make meditation a regular part of my life, I tend not to worry about things so much," and, "When I meditate, the atrocities in the world don't weigh me down as greatly." It's not that one ends up caring less. It is that one's communication, one's connection, is directly with The Divine, the Source, with That which lies beyond worldly events and concerns, not filtered by the ego. In deeper states of meditation, the ripples of the mind, that is thoughts themselves, are quieted. That is when the ever-present light of the Self, of the God that we are *all* one with, becomes visible. Such an experience automatically changes one's perceptions and motives. Such an encounter leads to true freedom.

The greatest paradigm shift possible is for people of service to act from that well of love which automatically arises when they live in the awareness of the connectedness of all things because of the light of The Divine. When we recognize and acknowledge that other beings in this world are but reflections of the same light, as we ourselves are, we can then see past *their* beliefs, arguments, judgments, and motives and realize that they have a purposeful life as well. Then and only then can our god be *the* God, the creator of all that is seen and unseen, the manifester who has come here to play billions of roles as billions of people. When the welfare of God's creation, i.e. the connectedness of all things, becomes priority one, all false gods fall into the fire: ego, money, materialism, ownership, superiority, importance, pride, insecurity, smallness, insignificance, and so on.

Those of us who have the amazing perspective which autism gives us are true gifts in this world. Those with limited vision will despise us for sure. But those with the ability to see past the illusory limitations will connect with us well. They will be our mentors. They will be our advocates. And we, in turn, will be forever grateful for their loving service and belief in us. They are the true heroes in this world. They give us the chance we need to shine our beacons outward so that we can connect with the Universe and with The Divine Presence that manifests as all. There is only one God, and we are it. Yes, all the world *is* a stage, and all the men and women merely players, as Shakespeare pointed out. Everyone is being played by the same Being, the universal and omnipresent Consciousness that sees through all our eyes simultaneously. Everything that is is, in fact, a Play of Consciousness.

20

Bringing It Home

By the summer of 2016, Becky and I were grounded enough financially and professionally that we decided it was time to make our life together permanent. We married in June during a backyard housewarming picnic. At the same point in time, my Aunt Doris, whom I spent a great deal of time with when I was a kid, felt as though her days on this earth were coming to an end because of her rapidly failing health. Therefore, she gave away all her money to me and my two brothers. She gave me a greater share because I was her godchild and because of recently getting married. Some of that money was immediately put toward filling a need I've been contemplating. I wanted to purchase a vehicle I could use as my actual office, something with enough headroom to stand up inside, space for my chiropractic table, and which had its own bathroom. It didn't take me long to find a used Class C motor home that fit my criteria perfectly. At the end of July, that then became my office which I used to travel around New Jersey. The down side was that driving such a large vehicle took some getting used to, and a lot of the money I made went into fixing it up and keeping it fueled. Therefore, I slowed things down a bit by reducing the number of zip codes I served to just 93.

That still encompassed much of the northwestern part of the state, though it eliminated most of the toll roads, run-down areas, and heavily congested areas as I had planned to do. As it got later into the year, it seemed only fitting that I start to wind things down in New Jersey altogether. After all, Christmas Eve was approaching, the day my twenty-month wait before being eligible to reactivate my PA license would be over. Although I thoroughly enjoyed what I did as a D.O.T. Medical Examiner, I desperately needed a break from all the hours upon hours and hundreds of miles of traveling in New Jersey. It was all taking a toll not just on the motor home but on me as well, both physically and mentally. It was time to conserve my energy so I could devote myself to being busy all over again closer to home after the new year. Besides, I was still new to the whole RVing thing, and I didn't want to be so far away in the event of extremely bad weather.

At about this same point in time, other professional changes were in the air. Becky was becoming exhausted and physically sick because of stress at her counseling job. Also, the efforts to remodel the loft above our garage came to a halt when our handyman found full-time work elsewhere and simply let our project sit. While it may seem as though we were taking one step forward and two steps back, an unexpected opportunity came along thanks to Matt, one of the U3: Body, Mind, & Spirit business partners. One of Matt's friends owned a building with a storefront that was scheduled to be available for rent in January. Matt brought this to the attention of Becky and the other business partner, Elizabeth, in hopes that this new development would revive our interest in creating another brick-and-mortar home for U3. U3 had been without one since leaving Kutztown in June 2014. The new building was located in Temple, right on a busy major roadway. The rental price was very affordable now that all four of us partners had viable incomes. Therefore, we jumped at the opportunity. We spent the first month of 2017 revamping the space, and during the first week in February U3 opened for business at its new location.

Finally, on February 8, 2017, I received my license to practice chiropractic in Pennsylvania. Now, for the first time since leaving my home town on November 14, 1992, I *finally* felt like I was home. I had a new wife and family, a new place to live, and now I could work in my own state. The circle was complete. Many life lessons, and much professional, personal, and spiritual evolution was endured over the years. Both time and my ASD/INFJ challenges proved that simply being in a certain role does not guarantee success. I never made an above-poverty-level income as an entrepreneur until 2016. I had lived below the poverty line for all but four of my adult years before then. The end of the funk brought about a new opportunity to stand tall and count my blessings. After all, one's success should never be measured by the amount of money he makes but by what he accomplishes in life. Holding onto this principle is difficult when you are facing homelessness and unfortunate transitions.

Soon after obtaining my license, Becky found a more fulfilling job doing exactly what she was already doing. Because of that, both her stress level and her physical health returned to normal. That just proved how being in the right environment among the right people can do so very much for how successful people become. One *needs* to be in a place where they feel appreciated and where they are rewarded for good work. It is also important to be where the opportunity for upward mobility is possible. As for me, once my Pennsylvania license went into effect, my Medical Examiner practice exploded beyond expectations because of the unfortunate passing of Dr. Tom O'Bierne, a fellow chiropractor who was also a mobile D.O.T. Medical

Examiner. I had listed myself in a total of 294 zip codes in southeastern PA, but I spent a great deal of time being listed as "unavailable" all due to the surprising influx of Dr. Tom's former patients.

Having faith that is strengthened by an unwavering connection to that which inspires you is vital to surviving. Also, patience is required — it's not just a virtue. Perseverance shows your true strength. God does help those who help themselves. Hiding from the world and simply calling it quits produces nothing, not even a possibility for success. Karma has treated me well because of my dedication to the spiritual path and because of my commitment to doing my work honestly. As Conan O'Brien said in his closing words during his final night as host of NBC's Tonight Show, "If you work really hard and you are kind, amazing things will happen." The work to be done is on improving your own outlook and demeanor. Kindness will always put you in the right situation eventually, even if you know you are being mistreated. It doesn't mean you surrender to being everyone's doormat. It *does* mean you recognize your own worth and advocate for yourself. The amazing results karma will determine and will present to you at the right time.

Bibliography

CHAPTER 1

1. Morgan Hill, "Homeless In America". *Demotix*. Corbis. Feb. 18, 2010. Web. December 17, 2014

2. http://autismworkbarrier.org.uk/articles/autism-homelessness-and-unemployment

3. Dr. Elizabeth Laugeson, assistant clinical professor at UCLA Semel Institute for Neuroscience & Human Behavior

CHAPTER 4

4. Nguyen, Thai, "How To Be The Nice Guy Who Never Finishes Last". Entrepreneur.com, Entrepreneur Media, Inc. March 4, 2015. Web. August 8, 2015.

CHAPTER 5

5. Bekiempis, Victoria, "The Anti-Vaccine Movement: A Brief History". *The Village Voice*. Village Media Group. July 26, 2012. Web. December 17, 2014

6. http://www.hrsa.gov/vaccinecompensation/data.html

7. http://www.cdc.gov/vaccines/vac-gen/additives.htm

8. Dorea, Jose, G. "Integrating Experimental (In Vitro and In Vivo) Neurotoxicity Studies of Low-dose Thimerosal Relevant to Vaccines". *Neurochemical Research*. June 2011, Volume 36, Issue 6, pp. 927-938

9. Faria, Jr., Miguel, A., M.D. "Vaccines (Part II): Hygiene, Sanitation, Immunization, and Pestilential Diseases". *Medical Sentinel*. Hacienda Publishing. March/April 2000. Volume 5, Issue #2

10. ibid

11. SV40 Cancer Foundation

12. Strickler, Howard. "Simian Virus 40 (SV40) and Human Cancers". *Einstein Quarterly Journal of Biology and Medicine*. (2001) 18:14-20

13. LaPoint, Terri. "Study Shows Link Between Autism And Vaccines Using Cells Lines From Aborted Babies". *The Inquisitr*. The Inquisitr News. November 2, 2014. Web. December 18, 2014

14. http://www.fda.gov/Drugs/ResourcesForYou/ Consumers/ucm289601.htm

15. Light, Donald W., Lexchin, Joel, Darrow, Jonathan J. "Institutional Corruption of Pharmaceuticals and the Myth of Safe and Effective Drugs". June 1, 2013. *Journal of Law, Medicine and Ethics*. American Society of Law, Medicine & Ethics, Inc. 2013, Vol. 14, No. 3: 590-610

16. http://teens.drugabuse.gov/drug-facts/prescription-drugs

17. Judith A. Lothian. Journal of Perinatal Education. 2009 Summer; 18(3): 48–54

18. http://www.mayoclinic.org/diseases-conditions/ high-blood-cholesterol/in-depth/statin-side-effects/ art-20046013

19. Texas Heart Institute Journal. 2006; 33(4): 417–423

20. Bowden, Johnny. "The Cholesterol Myth". *Better Nutrition.* Active Interest Media. July 2012. Web. Dec. 22, 2014

21. Eades, Michael, R., M.D. "Framingham Follies". *The Blog of Michael R. Eades, M.D.* September 26, 2006. Web. December 22, 2014

22. http://en.wikipedia.org/wiki/Statin

23. Siri-Tarino, et al. "Meta-analysis of prospective cohort studies evaluating the association of saturated fat with cardiovascular disease". *American Journal of Clinical Nutrition.* 2010 Mar;91(3):535-46. American Society for Nutrition. Article. June 27, 2017.

24. Sacks, Frank, et al. "Dietary Fats and Cardiovascular Disease: A Presidential Advisory From the American Heart Association". *Circulation.* June 15, 2017. American Heart Association. Article accessed June 27, 2017.

25. http://psychology.ucdavis.edu/faculty_sites/rainbow/html/facts_mental_health.html

26. Humphries, Suzanne, M.D. "Smoke, Mirrors, and the "Disappearance" Of Polio". *International Medical Council on Vaccinations*. November 17, 2011. International Medical Council on Vaccinations. Web. December 23, 2014

27. http://www.cdc.gov/vaccines/pubs/pinkbook/polio.html

28. Heasley, Shaun. "Autism Surge Due To Diagnostic Changes, Analysis Finds". *Disability Scoop*. June 29, 2012. Disability Scoop, LLC. Web. December 23, 2014

29. ibid

30. Wolinsky, Howard. "Disease Mongering and Drug Marketing". *EMBO Reports*. July 2005; 6(7): 612–614. EMBO Press. Web. December 23, 2014

31. ibid

32. ibid

CHAPTER 6

33. Tang, Guomei, et al. "Loss of mTOR-Dependent Macroautophagy Causes Autistic-like Synaptic Pruning Deficits". *Neuron*. Volume 83, Issue 5. March 9, 2014, pp. 1131-1143. Cell Press. Web. December 27, 2014

34. Hooker, Brian, S. "Measles-mumps-rubella vaccination timing and autism among young African American boys: a reanalysis of CDC data". *Translational Neurodegeneration*. August 27, 2014, 3:16. BioMed Central Ltd. Web. December 28, 2014

35. Rzhetsky, Andrey, et al. "Environmental and State-Level Regulatory Factors Affect the Incidence of Autism and Intellectual Disability". *PLOS Computational Biology*. March 13, 2014. Public Library of Science. Web. December 28, 2014

36. Goodman, Brenda. "Study: Factors Related to Oxygen Deprivation, Fetal Growth May Be Associated With Autism". *WebMD*. July 11, 2011. WebMD. Web. December 28, 2012

37. Shute, Nancy. "Scientists Implicate More Than 100 Genes In Causing Autism". *NPR.org*. October 29, 2014. National Public Radio. Web. December 28, 2014

38. Buie, Timothy. "The Relationship of Autism and Gluten". *Clinical Therapeutics*, Volume 35, Issue 5, pp. 578-583. May 2013. Elsevier Inc. Web. December 29, 2014

39. http://www.autismfile.com/science-research/ leaky-gut-and-autism

40. VaxXed: From Cover-up To Catastrophe, Directed by Andrew Wakefield, M.D., Produced by Autism Media Channel & Del Bigtree Productions, Released April 1, 2016

41. Samsel, Anthony & Seneff, Stephanie, "Glyphosate pathways to modern diseases V: Amino acid analogue of glycine in diverse proteins". *Journal of Biological Physics and Chemistry*. Volume 16, pp. 9-46. June 2016. Collegium Basilea & Association of Modern Scientific Investigation. Web. September 4, 2016.

42. http://www.momsacrossamerica.com/ glyphosate_testing_results . Accessed September 10, 2016.

43. http://www.momsacrossamerica.com/glyphosate_in_ childhood_vaccines . Accessed September 10, 2016

44. Towbin, Abraham, M.D. "Central nervous system damage in the human fetus and newborn infant: Mechanical and hypoxic injury incurred in the fetal-neonatal period". *American Journal of Diseases of Children*. June 1, 1970. American Medical Association. Volume 119, Issue 6, pp. 529-542. Web. December 29, 2014

45. Bisgaard, Hans, M.D., et al. "Cesarean Section and Chronic Immune Disorders". *Pediatrics*. 2015. Volume 135, Issue 1, pp. e92-e98. American Academy of Pediatrics. Web. April 3, 2016

46. Kassirer, Angell, M. "Alternative Medicine—the Risks of Untested and Unregulated Remedies". *New England Journal of Medicine*. 1998;339(12):839-841. Massachusetts Medical Society. Web. January 1, 2015

CHAPTER 7

47. Guzman, Timothy A. "Big Pharma and Big Profits: The Multibillion Dollar Vaccine Market". Global Research. Jan. 27, 2016. Centre for Research on Globalization. Web. October 23, 2016.

48. Miller, Neil Z. "Combining Childhood Vaccines At One Visit Is Not Safe". Journal of American Physicians and Surgeons. Volume 21, Number 2, Summer 2016, pp. 47-49. Association of American Physicians and Surgeons. Article. July 24, 2016.

49. Wells, Robert, D. " Non-B DNA conformations, Mutagenesis and disease". *Trends in Biochemical Sciences*. June 2007. Volume 32, Issue 6, pp. 271-278. Elsevier Trends Journals. Web. February 10, 2015.

50. http://www.fda.gov/BiologicsBloodVaccines/Vaccines/ApprovedProducts/ucm276859.htm

CHAPTER 8

51. Sharpless, Seth, K. "Susceptibility of spinal roots to compression block". *The Research Status of Spinal Manipulative Therapy*. NINCDS monograph 15, DHEW publication (NIH) 76-998:155, 1975.

52. Palmer, David, D. *The Science, Art, and Philosophy of Chiropractic*. P. 19. Portland Printing House Company. 1910.

53. Harrer, G, et al. " Comparison of equivalence between the St. John's Wort extract LoHyp-57 and fluoxetine". *Arzneimittel-Forschung*. Volume 49, Issue 4, pp. 289-286. April 1999. Thieme Medical Publishers, Inc. Web. January 3, 2015.

54. Crawford, Stephen, E., et al. " Using Reiki to decrease memory and behavior problems in mild cognitive impairment and mild Alzheimer's disease". *Journal of Alternative and Complementary Medicine*. Volume 12, Issue 9, pp. 911-913. November 2006. Mary Ann Liebert, Inc. Web. January 3, 2015

CHAPTER 10

55. http://www.16personalities.com/infj-relationships-dating

CHAPTER 15

56. http://education.jhu.edu/PD/newhorizons/ Exceptional%20Learners/Autism/Articles/Inclusion% 20of%20Students%20with%20Autism%20Spectrum% 20Disorders/

57. Sally Lindsay, Meghann Proulx, Helen Scott, Nicole Thomson. "Exploring teachers' strategies for including children with autism spectrum disorder in mainstream classrooms". *International Journal of Inclusive Education*. Vol. 18, Iss. 2, 2014, Taylor & Francis Group. Web. May 16, 2016

58. McKenna, Laura. "Boosting Social Skills in Autistic Kids With Drama". *The Atlantic*. June 1, 2016. Atlantic Media Company. Web. July 22, 2016

CHAPTER 16

59. Thornton, Shawnee. "Yoga for Improving Behavior in Children with Autism". *Yoga Digest*. April 2, 2015. Yoga Digest, LLC. Web. April 4, 2015

CHAPTER 18

60. http://www.gallup.com/products/170957/clifton-strengthsfinder.aspx